EFT for BACK PAIN

by Gary Craig

Emotional Freedom Techniques

www.emofree.com

Energy Psychology Press
P.O. Box 442, Fulton, CA 95439
www.energypsychologypress.com

Cataloging-in-Publication Data
Craig, Gary, 1940–
EFT for back pain / by Gary Craig and 59 EFT practitioners,
instructors, students, and users. — 1st ed.
  p. cm.
Includes index.
ISBN 978-1-60415-032-2
1. Backache—Alternative treatment. 1. Emotion-focused therapy.
I. Title.
RD771.B217C73 2009
617.5'6406—dc22

2009002944

Cover design by Victoria Valentine
Editing by CJ Puotinen
Typesetting by Karin Kinsey
Typeset in Cochin and Adobe Garamond
Printed in USA by Bang Printing
First Edition

10 9 8 7 6 5 4 3 2 1

Important note: While EFT (Emotional Freedom Techniques) has produced remarkable clinical results, it must still be considered to be in the experimental stage and thus practitioners and the public must take complete responsibility for their use of it. Further, Gary Craig is not a licensed health professional and offers EFT as an ordained minister and as a personal performance coach.

Contents

Acknowledgments

The list of individuals who contributed to the development of EFT can never be complete because most of them lived over 5,000 years ago. Those are the brilliant physicians who discovered and mapped the centerpiece of EFT, namely, the subtle energies that course through our bodies. These subtle energies are also the centerpiece of acupuncture and, as a result, EFT and acupuncture are cousins. Both disciplines are growing rapidly here in the West and, as time unfolds, they are destined to have a primary role in emotional and physical healing.

In the 20th Century, other dedicated souls advanced our use of ancient techniques that utilize the body's energy. Principal among them is Dr. George Goodheart, who developed Applied Kinesiology, a forerunner of EFT. In the 1960s, Dr. Goodheart discovered that muscle testing could be used to gather important information from the body, and he went on to train many health care practitioners and publish important books and papers.

Dr. John Diamond's work deserves applause because, to my knowledge, he was one of the first psychiatrists to use and write about these subtle energies. His many pioneering concepts, together with advanced ideas from Applied Kinesiology, have formed the foundation upon which our work is constructed. Dr. Diamond's best-sellers include *Life Energy: Using the Meridians to Unlock the Power of Your Emotions* (Continuum International, 1990) and *Life Energy and the Emotions* (Eden Grove, 1997).

Dr. Roger Callahan, the clinical psychologist from whom I received my original introduction to "emotional acupressure," deserves all the credit history can give him. He was the first to bring these techniques to the public in a substantial way and he did so despite open hostility from his own profession. As you might appreciate, it takes heavy doses of conviction to plow through the ingrained beliefs of conventional thinking.

Without Roger Callahan's missionary drive, we might still be sitting around theorizing about this "interesting thing."

It is upon the shoulders of these giants that I humbly stand. My own contribution to the rapidly expanding field of meridian therapies has been to reduce the unnecessary complexity that inevitably finds its way into new discoveries. EFT is an elegantly simple version of these procedures, which professionals and laypeople alike can use on a variety of problems.

I also owe a special debt of gratitude to Adrienne Fowlie, who, through a friend, introduced me to meridian tapping techniques and helped me develop EFT.

Many EFT students and practitioners helped make this book possible. I am grateful to all who contributed case studies and reports. Many of the examples given here were published in our email newsletter and are posted in the newsletter's archives on the EFT website, www.emofree.com.

The names given in the reports presented here have often been changed to protect the privacy of those involved. This is especially likely if only first names are given. All of the names given here are as they originally appeared in reports published in our newsletter and on the EFT website. When a person's full name is given, it has not been changed and is used with permission.

In the interests of editorial consistency, reports from the United Kingdom, Australia, Canada, and other countries that use British spelling and punctuation have been changed to conform to standard American English.

Like most topics of special interest, EFT has its own words and abbreviations that have special meaning for its students and practitioners. You'll find a list of EFT terms and their definitions in the Glossary at the end of this book.

Gary Craig

Introduction

This book—and the Emotional Freedom Techniques (EFT) it describes—will open your eyes to a new way of health and healing. It will most likely alleviate your back pain and keep it from ever returning while simultaneously improving your love life, your finances, your golf game, and your personal happiness. I know that sounds like hype from an infomercial. But it's true. EFT can do all of these things and more.

EFT's basic premise is that *the cause of all negative emotions is a disruption in the body's energy system.* I can't emphasize this concept enough. When our energy is flowing normally, without obstruction, we feel good in every way. When our energy becomes blocked or stagnant or is otherwise disrupted, negative or damaging emotions can develop along with all types of physical symptoms, including back pain.

EFT is often called *emotional acupuncture* because when you combine gentle tapping on key acupuncture points while focusing your thoughts on past events, present problems, physical discomfort, or anything else, the underlying emotional factors that contribute in any way to the situation are released along with the energy blocks along the acupuncture meridians.

Consider that:

- **EFT often relieves pain where nothing else will.**

- **Further, it brings relief in 80 percent of the cases in which it's tried,** and in the hands of a skilled practitioner, its success rate can exceed 95 percent.

- **Sometimes the pain goes away permanently** while in other cases the process needs to be continued. But even if pain returns, it can usually be reduced or eliminated quickly and effectively just by repeating the procedure.

- **People are often astonished at the results they experience** because their belief systems have not yet adapted to this common-sense process. Somehow, pain relief is supposed to be much more difficult than tapping with your fingertips on key acupuncture points.

- **EFT is extremely easy to use.** Small children learn it quickly, and kids as young as eight or ten have no trouble teaching it to others. It's fully portable, requires no special equipment, and can be used at any time of the day or night and under any circumstances.

- **No drugs, surgeries, radiations, or other medical interventions** are involved in EFT. In fact, it's so different from conventional medicine that the medical profession has no way of explaining its results.

- **It doesn't seem to matter what the patient's X-rays, blood tests, MRIs, CAT scans, or other diagnostic tests show.** Pain relief is likely to occur with EFT no matter what your diagnosis. That's because we are addressing a cause for pain that is outside the medical box.

- **This is not to say you should ignore your physician's advice.** On the contrary, I encourage you to consult with qualified health care providers. Quite a few EFT practitioners are physicians, nurses, dentists, acupuncturists, chiropractors, massage therapists, psychologists, counselors, and other health care providers. As EFT becomes more widely known, it will become easier to find licensed health care practitioners who are knowledgeable about EFT.

- **Using a few minutes of EFT will often end your pain for good.** When it doesn't, there is likely to be some underlying emotional issue that is creating chemicals and/or tension in your body that aggravates the pain.

- If that's the case, **EFT is ideal for collapsing and neutralizing emotional issues** and it often does the job in minutes. EFT was originally designed for reducing the psychotherapy process from months or years down to minutes or, in complicated cases, a few sessions.

What excites me most about EFT is its application to physical health and wellness. I'm convinced more than ever that Modern Medicine has walked right by a major contributor to chronic and acute diseases. Our unresolved angers, fears, and traumas show up in our physical bodies and manifest not just as back pain but as rheumatoid arthritis, cancer, multiple sclerosis, Parkinson's disease, and hundreds of other illnesses.

Just about everyone knows this intuitively. Whenever Los Angeles physician Eric Robins, MD, shows patients how to do EFT, he explains that past traumas can be stored in muscles and organs in the body and that releasing past events and all the emotions they generate may alleviate physical symptoms. Dr. Robins reports that most patients grasp this concept at once, and as soon as they tap away their anger, frustration, or unhappy memories, their symptoms improve.

Psychologists have always known that there are powerful connections between mind and body, but conventional talk therapy seldom cures anything, and neither do psychoactive drugs.

But balancing the body's energy can help with everything, and it's as simple as tapping on your head and torso while focusing on the problem. As Dr. Robins explains, this simple procedure releases or neutralizes the illness's underlying cause, and as soon as that happens, the illness itself disappears.

No technique or procedure works for everyone, but by all accounts, the vast majority of those who try EFT for a specific problem experience significant results. That's a stunning result, one that would be the envy of any prescription drug, surgical procedure, or medical treatment.

EFT has come a long way in the last ten years, but it's not even a blip on conventional medicine's radar. When it is noticed, it's often relegated to the "support therapy" category, something to be used later, after conventional treatments. I hope that will soon change. Unless there is a medical emergency that requires immediate attention, EFT should be the FIRST treatment offered. This, in my observation, will dramatically reduce the need for drugs, surgery, radiation, or other conventional procedures. Even in emergencies, such as accidents or injuries, EFT can be extremely helpful, for it helps people think clearly while reducing pain and discomfort. In all situations, it speeds recovery and healing.

To satisfy my curiosity about EFT's effectiveness in the treatment of serious diseases, I recently spent two years traveling to different cities giving three-day seminars in which I worked onstage with actual patients. As a result, I know more than ever that EFT is a truly universal healing tool. The same basic approach that treats back pain, diabetes, chronic fatigue syndrome, and multiple chemical sensitivities works as well for glaucoma, muscular dystrophy, rheumatoid arthritis, asthma, allergies, pulled hamstring muscles, high blood pressure heart disease, and every other physical ailment you can name. And when it comes to fears, phobias, anger, and anxiety, EFT is in a class by itself.

EFT is so new that it's still evolving. I encourage practitioners and newcomers alike to experiment – to try it on everything, not just on your back pain. It makes sense that if your energy is balanced, everything inside and around you benefits.

Whether you are already familiar with EFT or are a Newbie (my affectionate term for newcomers), I am very pleased to share this book with you. I know without a doubt that EFT can help you take control of your health and happiness and that the instructions and recommendations given here can completely transform your life.

In a nutshell, EFT is an emotional version of acupuncture, except we don't use needles. Instead, we stimulate the acupuncture meridians by tapping on them with our fingertips. This often brings forth astonishing results that are likely beyond your expectations. The procedure is easy to learn, easy to use, and easy to share with others. You will learn the basics and more in this book.

EFT is good for everything. While this book focuses on EFT's use for back pain, I must emphasize *that back pain represents but a tiny fraction of EFT's long list of successes.* For example, EFT is good for pain and symptoms of all kinds and often works where nothing else will. It is also astonishingly useful for emotional issues of every type and reduces the typical psychotherapy process from months or years down to minutes or hours. Further, those wishing to improve their performance in sports, business, public speaking, or the bedroom will also find EFT a valuable aid.

This book is like an encyclopedia. It is so comprehensive that it could easily be considered an "EFT Encyclopedia for Back Pain." Most readers will not need to read it all, but every reader will want to keep it around as a priceless resource because it contains approaches and concepts that you will not find in other health-related books.

This book contains creative approaches written by many EFT experts. EFT is an "open source" healing tool that encourages experimentation. This means that we start with an easy-to-learn, simple procedure that works beautifully in the majority of cases. After that, anyone can experiment with the process and develop other refinements. Thus, for your expanded education, we are sprinkling within this book the opinions, refinements, and creative approaches of dozens of EFTers.

Depending on your interest level, previous experience, and individual response to EFT, there are several ways to read this book.

If you are a "Newbie," or newcomer to EFT, I hope you may wish to start at the beginning and read it all the way through. By the time you reach the end, you will have an excellent chance of being completely and permanently free from pain, in addition to having a thorough understanding of EFT and the ability to share this useful technique with friends and family.

If you're impatient to get started, go straight to my *Quick Start* section. The Quick Start walks you through basic EFT, which by itself has brought relief to thousands. If basic EFT eliminates all of your pain for good, congratulations. You're one of our famous "One-Minute Wonders" and you can get on with your life. If the pain doesn't completely go away or if it returns at a later time, the rest of this book provides all the assistance you need to improve your results and make the improvements last.

If you're interested in the background of EFT and some of the technical, scientific, or engineering explanations that I'm fond of sharing, download our free *EFT Manual* from the official EFT website, www.emofree.com. This book was designed as a companion to the *EFT Manual* and you'll learn something valuable from both.

For convenience, the manual is also available as a paperback book sold in retail bookstores and online. Look for *The EFT Manual* (EFT: Emotional Freedom Techniques) by Gary Craig, published by Energy Psychology Press, 2008.

If you're an experienced EFTer, peruse the Table of Contents and go where your curiosity and interest take you. One of my goals in writing this book is to provide as many interesting examples as possible, so that all of us —including EFT instructors and practitioners—can add to our repertoire of approaches and strategies for making EFT more effective and versatile.

Our DVDs are vital to your complete comprehension of EFT. I would like to emphasize that this book and the EFT Manual do not contain everything there is to know about EFT. For example, there is no substitute for the demonstrations on our DVDs, which show EFT in action in seminars conducted throughout the United States.

The DVDs offer many live demonstrations of pain relief, including back, hip, and shoulder pain. For a complete description of the contents of each DVD, go to www.emofree.com/EFTStore/ and click on "full details" for any of the collections.

Once you understand the basics by watching the first hour of the first DVD in our introductory set, you can simply tap along with an endless number of sessions designed for your use. While doing so, you will learn as you go, you'll be entertained, and, without much effort, you will collapse or neutralize issues that have until now interfered with your recovery.

As I like to remind everyone, there is more human drama, inspiration, and humor in our videotaped seminars than there is in any reality television show!

In the last ten years, EFT has become a global phenomenon. Our free manual, which has been translated by EFT practitioners into 19 languages, has been downloaded by over half a million people, and another 5,000 to 10,000 download it every month. While most EFT practitioners live in the United States, the United Kingdom, Australia, and Canada, the technique is being taught and used in dozens of countries around the world. If you'd like to study EFT in Arabic, Bulgarian, Czech, Danish, Dutch, Finnish, French, German, Greek, Gujarati (a language of India), Hungarian, Italian, Norwegian, Persian (Farsi), Polish, Portuguese (from Brazil), Russian, Slovenian, Spanish, or Turkish, simply download the manual in translation.

The manual was written before I realized or understood how effective EFT can be in the treatment of physical symptoms such as back pain. Accordingly, it stresses emotional healings and doesn't cover physical healings in the dramatic fashion in which they occur. Because the manual has proven to be such an effective teaching tool, I have decided to leave it as is rather than modify it to emphasize the treatment of physical symptoms. It is the emotional and energetic factors that we need to understand, and those are profusely illustrated in its pages while physical symptoms are only briefly mentioned. For example, only two of the original EFT Manual's case reports describe physical pain.

Case History #11 from EFT Manual—Physical Pain

Lea attended one of the workshops I did for hypnotherapy students. She told me before the workshop that she had a lot of tight muscles and physical pain. I walked her through EFT for relief of the pain around her neck and shoulders. It subsided within two minutes. About an hour into the three-hour workshop, I asked her if the pain in her neck and shoulders had come back. She said no and then said that the *rest of the pain in her body had subsided as well…*

This is an example of how we address one problem with EFT and discover that other healings occur along the way. In Lea's case, the relief we gave to her neck and shoulder pain spilled over to the rest of her body. We then did another round of EFT and the balance of the pain went away, and it stayed away for the rest of the workshop. Pain like this is often caused by emotional distress and that's why EFT can be so effective in addressing it. However, new emotional stresses may bring the pain back. If so, repeated uses of EFT will likely give relief.

Case History #12 from EFT Manual—Low Back Pain

Donna is another example along these lines. She, too, attended one of my workshops and had such severe lower back pain that she didn't think she could stay for the entire one-day workshop. *"I just can't sit that long,"* she said. I helped her with EFT and her back did not bother her for the entire day.

These examples hint at what's possible, but the full story of EFT as a treatment for back pain deserves a book of its own.

Please keep in mind that all of the EFT techniques, approaches, formulas, and procedures described here apply not only to back pain but to *all types of pain.* They work equally well on migraines and other headaches, joint pain, arthritis, broken bones, muscle sprains, bruises, fibromyalgia, carpal tunnel syndrome, sports injuries, eyestrain, foot pain, toothaches, menstrual cramps, and indigestion. These same methods also work on all aspects of emotional pain. It's no exaggeration to say that the more you use and practice EFT, the easier it will be to apply it to any type of pain or discomfort—quickly and with a minimum of effort.

Pain's Emotional Causes

Medical schools provide little or no training in understanding or treating the emotional causes of illness, disease, or discomfort. They just make an occasional reference to stress aggravating certain problems, and that's as far as they go.

Yet our emotions have a profound effect on our physical symptoms. We all know this intuitively. For example, if I threw a live rattlesnake in your lap, wouldn't you have an instant emotion—such as fear—that would pump major amounts of adrenaline throughout your body?

When you are angry, doesn't your blood pressure go up? Doesn't your heart pound faster? Don't the veins in your neck stand out? Doesn't your face flush? During sexual arousal—an emotion—doesn't your body change in profound ways? And don't negative emotions sometimes cause your stomach to tighten...your throat to constrict...your head to ache?

These are obvious everyday proofs that our emotions profoundly impact our bodies. Yet how do these clear causes for our various symptoms escape the medical profession? Why aren't energy and emotions the front-running candidates as causes of pain and disease?

Physicians are taught early on in their training that the brain produces a wide array of chemicals that depend on our emotional moods. In fact, our brains are often referred to by the medical folks as "the world's most prolific pharmacy."

Negative emotions produce buckets of "negative chemicals" that circulate throughout the body causing excess acidity, chemical imbalances, and the like. It doesn't take a genius to predict the effect on our health of this consistent barrage of chemical insults. It is like putting bad gas in our automobiles. The eventual breakdown is both predictable and inevitable.

Positive emotions, on the other hand, generate healing chemicals and serve to produce balance. Have you ever noticed that love, laughter, and joy tend to reduce pain? Perhaps you can now see why, as EFT moves our systems from negative to positive emotions, it often provides powerful healing.

With these thoughts in mind, we see that the cause of our physical pains and symptoms must include our negative emotions because, without them, the resulting chemical imbalances would not occur.

Yet, the medical folks approach this problem *as though the unwanted chemicals are the problem.* That's why they offer drugs—additional chemicals—to counteract the effects of the unwanted chemicals. To them, that is the solution.

However, these body chemicals are *not* the problem. They are instead *symptoms* of the problem, and common sense would suggest that long-term, lasting relief comes from addressing the *cause* (the negative emotions) and not the *symptoms* (the resulting chemicals). That's what this book is about.

I am privileged to count many dedicated physicians as my personal friends. I have endless respect for their many talents and superb training regarding the chemical nature of the body. Many medical discoveries are impressive indeed and my doctor friends have countless wonderments at their disposal.

But their approach is limited.

It focuses on chemistry and does little or nothing about the energetic and emotional causes of pain and disease. When, for example, was the last time your physician spent any quality time asking you about your anger, fear, trauma, grief, and the like? Doesn't he or she just prescribe drugs or other conventional treatments instead?

That is where EFT comes in.

My hope is that by seeing how other people improved their lives and their backs with EFT, you'll develop a new set of strategies for dealing with pain and every other challenge that comes your way.

Quick Start

I won't keep you in suspense. If your back is in pain and you want a head start, just follow these simple instructions. You'll perform the basic version of EFT, and your pain may disappear right away.

On a scale from 0-to-10, with 10 being the worst, how much does your back hurt? Make a mental note of this number, and also check your range of motion by gently moving in different directions. The pain scale rating and range of motion are your "before" picture. When you complete the following exercise, which should take less than two minutes, compare your results.

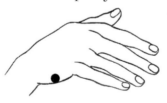

The Karate Chop (KC) Point

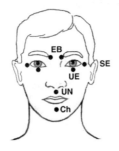

EB, SE, UE, UN and Ch Points

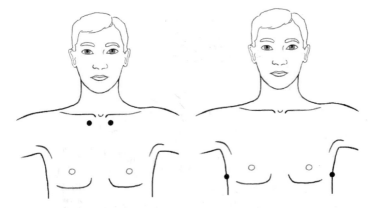

The Collarbone (CB) Points   The Underarm (UA) Points

Referring to the diagrams above, start tapping the side (KC = Karate Chop point) of one hand with the fingertips of the other hand while saying, *"Even though I have this pain in my back, I fully and completely accept myself."* Keep tapping while you say this statement three times. Say it whether or not you believe it. Belief is not required. Now move to your face and, using one or both hands, tap on all of the EFT points in sequence, moving down the body. Spend about seven taps on each point while you say the Reminder Phrase, *"Back pain."*

EB = Eyebrow — *"Back pain"*

SE = Side of Eye — *"Back pain"*

UE = Under Eye — *"Back pain"*

UN = Under Nose — *"Back pain"*

CH = Chin (under lip) — *"Back pain"*

CB = Collarbone — *"Back pain"*

UA = Under Arm — *"Back pain"*

Do this tapping sequence three times, tapping on each point approximately seven times as you move from Eyebrow to Under Arm.

When you finish, check your pain level. Has it stayed the same, gone up, or gone down? Has your range of motion changed? If you're like most people, you feel better already.

If your pain has completely disappeared, congratulations. You're done. You can get on with your life. If the pain comes back, or if you develop a new pain in your back, all you have to do is repeat the process.

If you feel better but still have some pain, tap on your Karate Chop point again but this time use the Setup Phrase, "Even though I still have some of this pain in my back, I fully and completely accept myself."

Keep tapping while you say this three times, then tap on the EFT points while saying, "This remaining pain." Complete the tapping sequence three times.

As before, check your progress by measuring your pain level and testing your range of motion. As long as you keep improving, this basic procedure will serve you well. You can repeat the sequence as often as needed. Thousands of people have reduced or eliminated their back pain in exactly this way.

If you still hurt, don't worry. This book describes many EFT techniques that are easy to learn and work fast.

Whether you stay with the basic formula or delve into EFT's exciting variations, this simple procedure can help you heal your back pain yourself.

1

EFT for Back Pain

Your back hurts, and you're not alone. At least 80 percent of all Americans suffer from back pain at some point in their lives, nearly 10 percent suffer from moderate to severe chronic pain, and an estimated 70 million are experiencing significant back pain right now, as you read this. Next to the common cold and upper respiratory infections, back pain is the leading cause of missed work days. Every year 200,000 Americans undergo spinal surgery in an effort to eliminate pain. In the United States alone, back pain costs almost 100 billion dollars per year in medical expenses. Back pain can turn strong people into invalids, destroy careers, wreck marriages, and cause a host of other problems.

According to medical experts, most cases of back pain are mechanical or non-organic, which means that they are not caused by illnesses such as inflammatory arthritis, infection, fractures, cancer, kidney stones, kidney disease, blood clots, or bone loss. Back pain can be a symptom of these and other diseases, but in most cases it is blamed on sprained ligaments, strained muscles, ruptured discs, irritated joints, repetitive motion injuries, slips, falls, trauma injuries, obesity, weak stomach muscles, overexertion, poor posture, improper lifting, sitting on a back-pocket wallet or billfold, sleeping on a bed that's too hard or too soft, sleeping next to a bedroom air conditioner, carrying a too-heavy back pack, alternating between sedentary and athletic activities, or simply being out of shape. You don't have to do anything dramatic to experience incapacitating back pain, either. Sometimes all it takes is a single sneeze or simply bending over to pick up a pencil.

Mark Grant, an Australian psychologist who specializes in managing chronic pain, says pain can be caused by muscle tension, changes in circulation, postural imbalances, psychological distress, and neurological damage. "It is also known," he says, "that unrelieved pain is associated with increased metabolic rate, spontaneous excitation of the central nervous system, changes in blood circulation to the brain, and changes in the limbic-hypothalamic system, the region of the brain that regulates emotions."

Acute and Chronic Pain

Acute back pain occurs suddenly. It's new. Chronic back pain is long-standing, permanent, or linked to old injuries.

Jennifer Schneider, MD, a specialist in pain management in Tucson, Arizona, says in her book *Living with Chronic Pain* (Healthy Living Books, Hatherleigh Press, 2004) that the nervous system is responsible for the two major types of chronic pain.

The first, called nociceptive pain, results from injury to muscles, tendons, ligaments, or internal organs. Undamaged nerve cells respond to a nearby injury by transmitting pain signals to the spinal cord and brain. The resulting pain is usually deep and throbbing, such as the pain from chronic low back problems, osteoarthritis, rheumatoid arthritis, fibromyalgia, headaches, interstitial cystitis, and chronic pelvic pain.

The second type of chronic pain, called neuropathic pain, results from abnormal nerve function or direct nerve damage. Damaged nerve fibers fire spontaneously at the injury site and along the nerve pathway, continuing even after the source of the injury has stopped sending pain messages. This type of pain can be constant or intermittent and is usually described as burning, aching, shooting, or stabbing. It sometimes radiates down the arms or legs. The medical conditions that contribute to neuropathic pain include shingles, diabetic neuropathy, reflex sympathetic dystrophy, phantom limb pain, radiculopathy, spinal stenosis, multiple sclerosis, Parkinson's disease, stroke, and spinal cord injuries.

"This type of pain," writes Dr. Schneider, "tends to involve exaggerated responses to painful stimuli, the spread of pain to areas that were not initially painful, and sensations of pain in response to normally non-painful stimuli, such light touch." It is often worse at night and may involve abnormal sensations such as tingling, pins and needles, or intense itching.

Some chronic pain syndromes involve both types of pain, such as sciatica, in which a pinched nerve causes back pain that radiates down the leg.

In addition, says Dr. Schneider, the consequences of chronic back pain typically extend well beyond the discomfort caused by pain sensations. Her list of potential physical effects includes poor wound healing, physical weakness, muscle breakdown, decreased movement that can lead to blood clots, shallow breathing and suppressed coughing that increase the risk of pneumonia, sodium and water retention in the kidneys, elevated heart rate and blood pressure, weakened immune system responses, a slowing of digestion and gastrointestinal motility, insomnia, loss of appetite and resulting weight loss, and increasing fatigue.

Those trapped in the vice of chronic back pain know that's only the beginning. As health columnist Jane Brody wrote in "Living with Pain That Just Won't Go Away" in the November 6, 2007, *New York Times*, "The psychological and social consequences of chronic pain can be enormous. Unremitting pain can rob a person of the ability to enjoy life, maintain important relationships, fulfill spousal and parental responsibilities, perform well at a job, or work at all.

"The economic burdens can be severe," she continues, "especially when the patient is the primary breadwinner or holds a job that provides the family's health insurance. Only about half of patients with chronic pain who undergo comprehensive multidisciplinary pain rehabilitation are able to return to work. As for the notion that chronic pain patients are often malingering – seeking attention and escape from responsibilities—pain specialists say that is nonsense. No one in his right mind—and most patients were in their right minds before the pain began—would trade a fulfilling life for the misery of chronic pain."

There are many medical treatments for acute and chronic back pain. Unfortunately, most of them have potentially adverse side effects and very few are considered cures. Even the most aggressive treatments, such as surgery, can have disappointing results, and the most innovative treatments can be prohibitively expensive, especially for those without adequate health insurance.

Because conventional medicine has such a dismal track record, many back pain sufferers have turned to alternative or complementary treatments such as chiropractic adjustments, acupuncture, acupressure, medicinal herbs, massage, postural alignment techniques, hydrotherapy, hypnosis, therapeutic yoga, core-conditioning exercise, aromatherapy, or other modalities, all of which have brought relief to many. Most of these require repeated treatments, which can be expensive and time-consuming. And these treatments don't always work, either. The pain may never improve, or it may go away and come back, or new injuries can trigger new waves of pain in the same old places.

Why can't the medical profession cure your back pain once and for all? I believe it's because modern medicine's goal is to suppress symptoms. That's what the term *allopathic*, which is used to describe conventional Western medicine, means. Allopathic physicians focus on symptoms such as spasms and inflammation, then prescribe drugs and other treatments that suppress them.

At no time do they search for the symptoms' underlying causes. As a result, physicians and the patients they treat are looking in the wrong place for answers. The true causes of back pain are not what most of us expect, *for the true causes don't have anything to do with slipped discs, strained muscles, or osteoarthritis.*

What causes chronic pain? To answer that important question, consider the discoveries of John E. Sarno, M.D. A professor of Rehabilitation Medicine at the New York University School of Medicine, Dr. Sarno is the author of three best-selling books about musculoskeletal pain, and his latest book, *The Divided Mind: The Epidemic of Mindbody Disorders* (HarperCollins, 2006), explores the many connections between our emotions and our health.

In a nutshell, Dr. Sarno says that your back hurts because you are angry. As soon as you realize that and find a way to release your anger, your back will stop hurting. This is why so many promising treatments for back pain don't work, or they work for a while but the pain keeps coming back. The underlying cause is still there, says Dr. Sarno—you're still angry—and so your body continues to generate pain.

Needless to say, Dr. Sarno's theory is controversial, but thousands of patients have responded to his treatment, and six highly regarded physicians who use his methods contributed chapters to *The Divided Mind*. Like Dr. Sarno, they believe that the only sensible way to approach back pain and other chronic conditions is by treating the emotional factors that cause physical symptoms.

That's my approach, too, but I go a step further and address the underlying causes of the anger that contributes to pain by combining acupressure with focused thought in EFT. Not only does this approach reduce or eliminate pain in minutes for about 80 percent of those who try it (which is, by the way, an incredible success rate for any health treatment), but in many cases the pain completely clears up in a very short time and stays away with no further treatment.

Larry Burk MD, a radiologist in North Carolina, appeared on one our DVDs and discussed these concepts with me at some length. Interestingly, he has seen many X-rays and MRIs wherein medical explanations are quite divergent from people's experiences of pain.

Pain and Emotions

by Larry Burk, MD

It is instructive to note that many ailments which seem to have an underlying anatomical cause may also have a deeper emotional root as well. As a radiologist, I am acutely aware of this situation since there are many scientific studies of MRI indicating that a surprising number of people with no symptoms whatsoever have rather dramatic abnormalities on scans obtained on a volunteer basis for research purposes. Equally puzzling, there are many patients with severe debilitating pain from conditions such as fibromyalgia who have no abnormalities on any MRI scans.

In 2001, David G. Borenstein, MD, published an article in *The Journal of Bone and Joint Surgery* entitled "The Value of Magnetic Resonance Imaging of the Lumbar Spine to Predict Low-Back Pain in Asymptomatic Subjects: A Seven-Year Follow-up Study." In 1989, a group of 67 asymptomatic individuals with no history of back pain underwent magnetic resonance imaging of the lumbar spine. Twenty-one subjects (31 percent) had an identifiable abnormality of a disc or of the spinal canal. The findings on magnetic resonance scans were not predictive of the development or duration of low-back pain.

Similar studies have been reported in asymptomatic volunteers for MRI findings in the cervical and thoracic spine, the shoulder, and the knee. This research calls into question the assumed cause-and-effect relationship between symptoms and anatomical abnormalities. The same issues are raised by the fact that some patients get better when their physical pathology is corrected through surgery, and some do not. In additional research studies on the placebo effect, sham surgery has produced relief of symptoms when nothing but a skin incision was made at the time of the procedure. All of this information lends support to the concept that deeper emotional issues are at the root, which can be addressed with EFT.

✴ ✴ ✴

To support the theory that pain is caused by anger and other negative emotions, here are some observations from Dr. Eric Robins, a Los Angeles physician and EFT practitioner.

Pain and Anger

by Eric Robins, MD

For decades, John Sarno, M.D., has seen the worst chronic pain patients in the world. Most lived with severe pain in the neck, back, shoulder, or buttocks for 10 to 30 years. Most received multiple epidural injections, one or more surgeries, and years of physical therapy. They all had terrible mechanisms of action, such as a forklift truck falling on them or a 747 jet rolling over them, and all their X-rays looked like the "Elephant Man." They all had a good reason for their pain.

Yet even with this challenging collection of patients, Dr. Sarno has a 70-percent cure rate with regard to both pain and function, and an additional 15 percent of his patients are much improved, typically 40 to 80 percent better. He has had these results with about 12,000 patients.

Typically when a pain patient goes to a physician for help, the doctor orders an MRI scan, which invariably shows some sort of anatomic abnormality like a slipped disc. The doctor concludes that the disc is causing the pain and prescribes symptom-suppressing drugs or therapies. Unfortunately, this approach usually has poor long-term results. The pain may disappear for a while, but it soon comes back, often worse than before.

Dr. Sarno looked at the medical literature and found an interesting study in the *New England Journal of Medicine*. It showed that if you take 100 middle-aged people who have *NO* back pain and do MRI scans on them, 65 percent will have a slipped disc or spinal stenosis. In other words, these people have conditions that are blamed for most of the world's back pain, yet they experience no pain at all. He began asking himself, "If the disc isn't causing this pain, then what is?"

What he discovered is that his pain patients had chronic tension and spasm of the muscles of the neck, back, shoulder, or buttocks. When a muscle is chronically tensed, the blood can't flow through it, resulting in a relative lack of oxygen, and this is what causes severe pain.

Then Dr. Sarno asked himself, "Why would someone have chronically tensed muscles to begin with?" He realized that many of us grow up learning, on an unconscious level, that it's not okay to feel or express our anger or anxiety.

The problem of course is that as we grow up, we experience many specific events or traumas that elicit anger or anxiety. As these emotions start to emerge, our unconscious mind basically says, "It's not okay or safe to be feeling these things." Then, Dr. Sarno explains, the unconscious mind causes muscles to clamp down and tighten in order to cause a pain that takes our minds off of what we are angry or anxious about.

Almost all of us, including most physicians, believe that pain serves a useful purpose, that it protects us from more serious damage or injury. In contrast,

Dr. Sarno quotes Stanley J. Coen of the Columbia University College of Physicians and Surgeons, who first suggested that psychosomatic physical symptoms were most likely a defense against harmful or toxic unconscious emotional phenomena. In other words, physical symptoms such as back pain are a reaction to unconsciously generated feelings that are repressed as a matter of self-preservation, Dr. Sarno discovered that simply becoming aware of these feelings can lead to a cure.

He obtained his amazing results by bringing folks in for two lectures. In the first lecture he'd tell them, "It's not the disc or spinal stenosis or any other anatomic abnormality that's causing your pain. Most people your age who have no pain have a slipped disc or spinal stenosis or other conditions that are normally blamed for back pain. What is causing your pain is chronic tension and spasm of the muscles."

In the second lecture he'd tell them, "Whenever you have pain, I want you to notice what you're angry or anxious about." Dr. Sarno then had his patients write in a journal, enroll in group therapy sessions, or engage in psychotherapy. He reported that about 20 percent of his patients weren't consciously aware of what they were angry or anxious about, and those patients needed to work with a therapist to get in touch with some repressed or unconscious material.

I explain Dr. Sarno's model whenever I speak to groups because he gets such amazing results, and of course the proof is in the pudding. In one of his books, he explains that this emotional model works not just for musculoskeletal pain; it can be used for most chronic or functional illnesses.

Dr. Sarno's discoveries are an important break-through, but the methods he recommends to handle emotional issues are archaic compared to the speed and efficiency of EFT. We can expect better and faster results by combining Dr. Sarno's insights with EFT, which is the best and fastest mind-body healing technique in clinical use in the world right now.

❊ ❊ ❊

In his busy clinical practice, Dr. Robins, who is a urologist, teaches EFT to patients whose symptoms don't respond to conventional treatment. He explains to them that we store trauma not only in our minds but in different parts of the body, including muscles, bones, and organs. Most patients grasp the idea immediately and offer suggestions as to what event, memory, or problem might be stored in their kidney or bladder or other problem area. In many cases, he has cancelled scheduled surgery or taken patients off of prescription drugs because they were no longer needed. .

If Dr. Sarno can produce such amazing results just by helping people intellectually understand the underlying causes of their pain, and if Dr. Robins can help his patients cure themselves just by demonstrating EFT in a busy clinic, imagine what you can do with a little time and practice using not only basic EFT but some of the most sophisticated, effective discoveries that are used by EFT practitioners. If you read this book all the way through, practice all the exercises, and experiment with all the scripts, you'll not only be well on your way to healing your back and saying goodbye to its pain, now and forever, but you'll be an expert on EFT and its art of delivery.

Using EFT

Are you ready to let your body heal itself? Let's get started.

Defining the problem

Your problem is back pain, but before you begin using EFT, take a moment to define your "before" picture. One way to do this is to rate your pain on a scale from 0-to-10. In EFT, we call this the Intensity Meter.

Measuring Intensity

0 – 1 – 2 – 3 – 4 – 5 – 6 – 7 – 8 – 9 – 10

none/mild discomfort/moderate discomfort/major discomfort/maximum pain

How does your back feel right now? If you have to be reminded that you're in pain, and when you look for it you remember that it's there, but only just a little, you're in the "mild discomfort" zone and you'll give it a 1, 2, or 3. If it's slightly more intense, so that you can still move around but you're consciously aware of the pain, it's a 4, 5, or 6. If the pain is a major discomfort, something you can't forget about and it interferes with your ability to move, it's a 7, 8, or 9. A pain that's the maximum you can endure, which is as bad as it gets, is a 10.

It's a good idea to rate every problem before and after you apply EFT so that you can determine how much progress you're making. Don't worry if you find it difficult to select a specific number – sometimes Newbies get distracted by this part of the procedure and worry about whether it's a 5 or a 6, or a 2 or a 3. Using the 10-point scale gets easier with practice. Just give yourself a number to get started and it will soon become automatic. For reference, jot the number down and add a few notes about where the pain is located, how it interferes with your range of motion, and whether it hurts more when you move to the left or right, stand or sit, and so forth.

Another way to indicate the intensity of your back pain is visually, by stretching your arms wide apart for major pain and putting them close together for minor pain. This method works well for children, who find it easier to express "big" and "small" with their hands than with a number scale.

Or you might visualize your pain as a thermometer, with the red line reaching the top for major pain and falling to the bottom for minor pain. Or you might visualize a meter that looks like a gas gauge, with minor pain at the zero or empty indicator on the left side and major pain on the 100 or full indicator on the right side.

The method you choose doesn't matter as long as it works for you. Keeping track of your pain's intensity before and after treatment is the easiest way to determine whether and how effectively the treatment is working.

Now, borrowing some pages from the EFT manual, I'd like to introduce you to the Basic Recipe, the formula that is the foundation of this technique.

The Basic Recipe

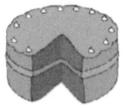

A recipe has certain ingredients which must be added in a certain order. If you are baking a cake, for example, you must use sugar instead of pepper and you must add the sugar *before* you put it in the oven. Otherwise… no cake.

Basic EFT is like a cake recipe. It has specific ingredients that go together in a specific way. Just as someone who is learning to cook will get best results from following tried and true instructions, someone who is new to EFT will do well to learn the basic recipe. An accomplished chef will take a different approach, and so can you once you master the fundamentals.

Although I am going to some length to describe it in detail, the Basic Recipe is very simple and easy to do. *Once memorized, each round of it can be performed in about one minute.* It will take some practice, of course, but after a few tries the whole process will becomes so familiar that you can bake that emotional freedom cake in your sleep. You will then be well on your way to mastery of EFT and all the rewards it provides.

Let me interject here that various shortcuts are available and described later in this book and in our DVDs. I am describing the *full* Basic Recipe here because it provides an important foundation to the whole process. The proficient practitioner may want to use the shortcuts because they cut the average time involved by at least half.

The full Basic Recipe consists of four ingredients, two of which are identical. They are:

1. The Setup

2. The Sequence

3. The 9 Gamut Procedure

4. The Sequence (again)

Ingredient #1: The Setup

Applying the Basic Recipe is something like going bowling. In bowling, there is a machine that sets up the pins by picking them up and arranging them in perfect order at the end of the alley. Once this "setup" is done, all you need to do is roll the ball down the alley to knock over the pins.

In a similar manner, the Basic Recipe has a beginning routine to "set up" your energy system as though it was a set of bowling pins. This routine (called the Setup) is vital to the whole process and prepares the energy system so that the rest of the Basic Recipe (the ball) can do its job.

Your energy system, of course, is not *really* a set of bowling pins. It is a set of subtle electric circuits. I present this bowling analogy only to give you a sense for the purpose of the Setup and the need to make sure your energy system is properly oriented before attempting to remove its disruptions.

Your energy system is subject to a form of electrical interference which can block the balancing effect of these tapping procedures. When present, this interfering blockage must be removed or the Basic Recipe will not work. Removing it is the job of the Setup.

Technically speaking, this interfering blockage takes the form of a *polarity reversal* within your energy system. This is *not* the same thing as the *energy disruptions* which cause your negative emotions.

Another analogy may help us here. Consider a flashlight or any other device that runs on batteries. If the batteries aren't there, it won't work. Equally important, *the batteries must be installed properly*. You've noticed, I'm sure, that batteries have + and - marks on them. Those marks indicate their *polarity*. If you line up those + and - marks according to the instructions, then the electricity flows normally and your flashlight works fine.

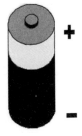

But what happens if you put the batteries in backwards? Try it sometime. The flashlight will not work. It acts as if the batteries have been removed. That's what happens when polarity reversal is present in your energy system. It's like your batteries are in backwards. I don't mean you stop working altogether...like turn "toes up" and die...but your progress *does* become arrested in some areas.

This polarity reversal has an official name. It is called Psychological Reversal and it represents a fascinating discovery with wide-ranging applications in...*all areas of healing and personal performance.*

It is the reason why some diseases are chronic and respond very poorly to conventional treatments. It is also the reason why some people have such a difficult time losing weight or giving up addictive substances. It is, quite literally, the cause of self-sabotage.

Psychological Reversal is caused by self-defeating, negative thinking which often occurs subconsciously and thus outside of your awareness. On average, it will be present—and thus hinder EFT—about 40 percent of the time. Some people have very little of it (this is rare) while others are beset by it most of the time (this also is rare). Most people fall somewhere in between these two extremes. Psychological reversal doesn't create any feelings within you so you won't know if it is present or not. Even the most positive people are subject to it....including yours truly.

When psychological reversal is present, it will stop any attempt at healing, including EFT, dead in its tracks. Therefore…*it must be corrected if the rest of the Basic Recipe is going to work.*

Being true to the 100-percent overhaul concept, we correct for Psychological Reversal *even though it might not be present.* It only takes 8 or 10 seconds to do and, if it isn't present, no harm is done. If it *is* present, however, a major impediment to your success will be out of the way.

That being said, here's how the Setup works. There are two parts to it…

You repeat an affirmation three times while you rub the "Sore Spot" or, alternatively, tap the "Karate Chop" point (these will be explained shortly).

The Affirmation

Since the cause of Psychological Reversal involves negative thinking, it should be no surprise that the correction for it includes a neutralizing affirmation. Such is the case and here it is.

Even though I have this _____, I deeply and completely accept myself.

The blank is filled in with a brief description of the problem you want to address. Here are some examples.

Even though I have this <u>pain in my lower back</u>, I deeply and completely accept myself.

Even though I have this <u>fear of public speaking</u>, I deeply and completely accept myself.

Even though I have this <u>headache</u>, I deeply and completely accept myself.

Even though I have this <u>anger towards my father</u>, I deeply and completely accept myself.

Even though I have this <u>war memory</u>, I deeply and completely accept myself.

Even though I have this <u>stiffness in my neck</u>, I deeply and completely accept myself.

Even though I have <u>these nightmares</u>, I deeply and completely accept myself.

Even though I have this <u>craving for alcohol</u>, I deeply and completely accept myself.

Even though I have this <u>fear of snakes</u>, I deeply and completely accept myself.

Even though I have this <u>depression</u>, I deeply and completely accept myself.

This is only a partial list, of course, because the possible issues that are addressable by EFT are endless. You can also vary the acceptance phrase by saying:

"I accept myself even though I have this _____ _____."

"Even though I have this _____, I deeply and profoundly accept myself."

"I love and accept myself even though I have this _____."

All of these affirmations are correct because they follow the same general format. That is, they acknowledge the problem and create self acceptance despite the existence of the problem.

That is what's necessary for the affirmation to be effective. You can use any of them but I suggest you use the recommended one because it is easy to memorize and has a good track record at getting the job done.

Now here are some interesting points about the affirmation.

It doesn't matter whether you believe the affirmation or not...just say it.

It is better to say it with feeling and emphasis, but saying it routinely will usually do the job.

It is best to say it out loud, but if you are in a social situation where you prefer to mutter it under your breath, or do it silently, then go ahead. It will probably be effective.

To add to the effectiveness of the affirmation, the Setup also includes the simultaneous rubbing of a "Sore Spot" or tapping on the "Karate Chop" point. They are described next.

The Sore Spot

There are two Sore Spots and it doesn't matter which one you use. They are located in the upper left and right portions of the chest and you find them as follows:

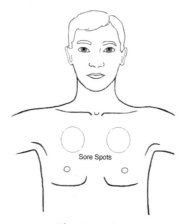

The Sore Spot

Go to the base of the throat about where a man would knot his tie. Poke around in this area and you will find a U shaped notch at the top of your sternum (breastbone). From the top of that notch go down 2 or 3 inches toward your navel and then 2 or 3 inches to your left (or right). You should now be in the upper left (or right) portion of your chest. If you press vigorously in that area (within a 2-inch radius) you will find a "Sore Spot." This is the place you will need to rub while saying the affirmation.

This spot is usually sore or tender when you rub it vigorously because lymphatic congestion occurs there. When you rub it, you are dispersing that congestion. Fortunately, after a few episodes the congestion is all dispersed and the soreness goes away. Then you can rub it with no discomfort whatsoever.

I don't mean to overplay the soreness you may feel. It's not like you will have massive, intense pain by rubbing this Sore Spot. It is certainly bearable and should cause no undue discomfort. If it does, then lighten up your pressure a little.

Also, if you've had some kind of operation in that area of the chest or if there's any medical reason whatsoever why you shouldn't be probing around in that specific area then *switch to the other side.* Both sides are equally effective. In any case, if there is any doubt, consult your health practitioner before proceeding or tap the Karate Chop point instead.

The Karate Chop Point

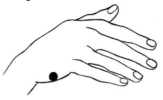

The Karate Chop (KC) Point

The Karate Chop point (abbreviated **KC**) is located at the center of the fleshy part of the outside of your hand (either hand) between the top of the wrist and the base of the baby finger or, stated differently, the part of your hand you would use to deliver a karate chop.

Instead of rubbing it as you would the Sore Spot, you vigorously *tap* the Karate Chop point with the fingertips of the index finger and middle finger—or all fingers—of the other hand. While you *could* use the Karate Chop point of either hand, it is usually most convenient to tap the Karate Chop point of the non-dominant hand with the fingertips of the dominant hand. If you are right-handed, tap the Karate Chop point on the left hand with the fingertips of the right hand. If you are left-handed, tap the Karate Chop point on your right hand with the fingertips of your left hand.

Should you use the Sore Spot or the Karate Chop point? After years of experience with both methods, it has been determined that rubbing the Sore Spot is a bit more effective than tapping the Karate Chop point. It doesn't have a commanding lead by any means but it *is* preferred.

Because the Setup is so important in clearing the way for the rest of the Basic Recipe to work, I urge you to use the Sore Spot rather than the Karate Chop point. It puts the odds a little more in your favor. However, the Karate Chop point is perfectly useful and will clear out any interfering blockage in the vast majority of cases. So feel free to use it if the Sore Spot is inappropriate for any reason.

You will notice that in our videotaped seminars, I often instruct people to tap the Karate Chop point instead of rub the Sore Spot. That's because it is easier to teach when I'm on stage.

Now that you understand the parts to the Setup, performing it is easy. You create a word or short phrase to fill in the blank in the affirmation and then...simply repeat the affirmation, with emphasis, three times while continuously rubbing the Sore Spot or tapping the Karate Chop point.

That's it. After a few practice rounds, you should be able to perform the Setup in 8 seconds or so. Now, with the Setup properly performed, you are ready for the next ingredient in the Basic Recipe...The Sequence.

Ingredient #2: The Sequence

The Sequence is very simple in concept. It involves tapping on the end points (key acupooints) of the major energy meridians in the body and is the method by which the "zzzzzt" in the energy system is balanced out. Before locating these points for you, however, you need a few tips on how to carry out the tapping process.

Tapping Tips:

- You can tap with either hand but it is usually more convenient to do so with your dominant hand (your right hand if you are right-handed or your left hand if you are left-handed).

- Tap with the fingertips of your index finger and middle finger. This covers a little larger area than just tapping with one fingertip and allows you to cover the tapping points more easily.

- Tap solidly but never so hard as to hurt or bruise yourself.

- Tap about seven times on each of the tapping points. I say about seven times because you will be repeating a "reminder phrase" (covered later) while tapping and it will be difficult to count at the same time. If you are a little over or a little under seven (five to nine, for example) that will be sufficient.

Most of the tapping points exist on either side of the body. It doesn't matter which side you use nor does it matter if you switch sides during The Sequence. For example, you can tap under your right eye and, later in The Sequence, tap under your left arm.

The points: Each energy meridian has two end points. For the purposes of the Basic Recipe, you need only tap on one end to balance out any disruptions that may exist in it. These end points are near the surface of the body and are thus more readily accessed than other points along the meridians that may be more deeply buried. What follows are instructions on how to locate the end points of those meridians that are important to the Basic Recipe. Taken together...and done in the order presented...they form The Sequence.

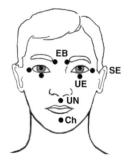

EB, SE, UE, UN and Ch Points

Eyebrow: At the beginning of the eyebrow, just above and to one side of the nose. This point is abbreviated **EB** for beginning of the EyeBrow.

Side of Eye: On the bone bordering the outside corner of the eye. This point is abbreviated **SE** for Side of the Eye.

Under Eye: On the bone under an eye about 1 inch below your pupil. This point is abbreviated **UE** for Under the Eye.

Under Nose: On the small area between the bottom of your nose and the top of your upper lip. This point is abbreviated **UN** for Under the Nose.

Chin: Midway between the point of your chin and the bottom of your lower lip. Although it is not directly on the point of the chin, we call it the chin point because it is descriptive enough for people to understand easily. This point is abbreviated **Ch** for Chin.

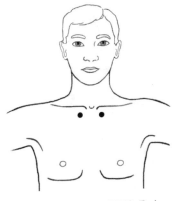

The Collarbone (CB) Points

Collarbone: The junction where the sternum (breast-bone), collarbone and first rib meet. Place your forefinger on the U-shaped notch at the top of the breastbone (where a man would knot his tie). Move down toward the navel 1 inch and then go to the left (or right) 1 inch. This point is abbreviated **CB** for CollarBone *even though it is not on the collarbone (or clavicle) per se.* It is at the *beginning* of the collarbone.

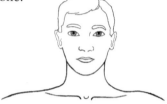

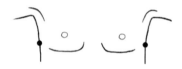

The Underarm (UA) Points

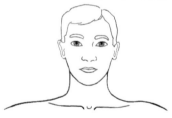

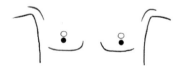

The Below Nipple (BN) Points

Underarm: On the side of the body, at a point even with the nipple (for men) or in the middle of the bra strap (for women). It is about 4 inches below the armpit. This point is abbreviated **UA** for Under the Arm.

Below Nipple: For men, one inch below the nipple. For ladies, where the underskin of the breast meets the chest wall. This point is abbreviated **BN** for Below Nipple.

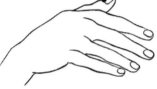

The Thumb (Th) Point

Thumb: On the outside edge of your thumb at a point even with the base of the thumbnail. This point is abbreviated **Th** for Thumb.

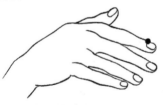

The Index Finger (IF) Point

Index Finger: On the side of your index finger (the side facing your thumb) at a point even with the base of the fingernail. This point is abbreviated **IF** for Index Finger.

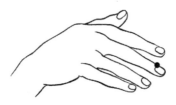

The Middle Finger (MF) Point

Middle Finger: On the side of your middle finger (the side closest to your thumb) at a point even with the base of the fingernail. This point is abbreviated **MF** for Middle Finger.

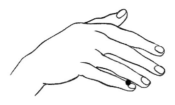

The Baby Finger (BF) Point

Baby Finger: On the inside of your baby finger (the side closest to your thumb) at a point even with the base of the fingernail. This point is abbreviated **BF** for Baby Finger.

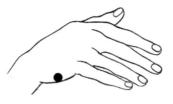

The Karate Chop (KC) Point

Karate Chop: The last point is the karate chop point... which has been previously described under the section on the Setup. It is located in the middle of the fleshy part on the outside of the hand between the top of the wrist bone and the base of the baby finger. It is abbreviated **KC** for Karate Chop.

The abbreviations for these points are summarized below in the same order as given above.

EB = Beginning of the **E**ye**B**row

SE = **S**ide of the **E**ye

UE = **U**nder the **E**ye

UN = **U**nder the **N**ose

Ch = **Ch**in

CB = Beginning of the **C**ollar**B**one

UA = **U**nder the **A**rm

BN = **B**elow the **N**ipple

Th = **Th**umb

IF = **I**ndex **F**inger

MF = **M**iddle **F**inger

BF = **B**aby **F**inger

KC = **K**arate **C**hop

Please notice that these tapping points proceed *down the body*. That is, each tapping point is *below* the one before it. That should make it a snap to memorize. A few trips through it and it should be yours forever.

Also note that the BN point has been added since the making of our introductory DVDs It was originally left out because it was awkward for ladies to tap while in social situations (restaurants, etc.). Even though the EFT results have been superb without it, I include it now for completeness.

Ingredient #3: The 9 Gamut Procedure

The 9 Gamut Procedure is, perhaps, the most bizarre looking process within EFT. Its purpose is to "fine tune" the brain and it does so via some eye movements and some humming and counting. Through connecting nerves, certain parts of the brain are stimulated when the eyes are moved. Likewise the right side of the brain (the creative side) is engaged when you hum a song and the left side (the digital side) is engaged when you count.

The 9 Gamut Procedure is a 10-second process in which nine "brain-stimulating" actions are performed while continuously tapping on one of the body's energy points...the Gamut point. It has been found, after years of experience, that this routine can add efficiency to EFT and hastens your progress towards emotional free-dom...especially when *sandwiched* between 2 trips through The Sequence.

One way to help memorize the Basic Recipe is to look at it as though it was a ham sandwich. the Setup is the preparation for the ham sandwich and the sandwich itself consists of two slices of bread (the Sequence) with the ham, or middle portion, as the 9 Gamut Procedure. It looks like this.

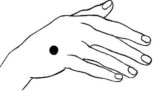

The Gamut Point

To do the 9 Gamut Procedure, you must first locate the Gamut point. It is on the back of either hand and is 1/2 inch behind the midpoint between the knuckles at the base of the ring finger and the little finger.

If you draw an imaginary line between the knuckles at the base of the ring finger and little finger and consider that line to be the base of an equilateral triangle whose other sides converge to a point (apex) in the direction of the wrist, then the gamut point would be located at the apex of the triangle.

Next, you must perform nine different actions while tapping the Gamut point continuously. These 9 Gamut actions are:

1. Eyes closed.

2. Eyes open.

3. Eyes hard down right while holding the head steady.

4. Eyes hard down left while holding the head steady.

5. Roll eyes in a circle as though your nose is at the center of a clock and you are trying to see all the numbers in order.

6. Roll eyes in a circle in the reverse direction.

7. Hum two seconds of a song (I usually suggest "Happy Birthday").

8. Count rapidly from 1 to 5.

9. Hum two seconds of a song again.

Note that these nine actions are presented in a certain order and I suggest that you memorize them in the order given. However, you can mix the order up if you wish so long as you do all nine of them...*and*...you perform the last three together as a unit. That is, you hum for two seconds, then count, then hum the song again, in that order. Years of experience have proven this to be important.

Also, note that for some people humming "Happy Birthday" causes resistance because it brings up memories of unhappy birthdays. In this case, you can either use EFT on those unhappy memories and resolve them... *or*...you can side-step this issue for now by substituting some other song.

Ingredient #4: The Sequence (again)

The fourth and last ingredient in the Basic Recipe was mentioned above. It is an identical trip through the Sequence.

The Reminder Phrase

Once memorized, the Basic Recipe becomes a lifetime friend. It can be applied to an almost endless list of emotional and physical problems and provides relief from most of them. However, there's one more concept we need to develop before we can apply the Basic Recipe to a given problem. It's called the Reminder Phrase.

When a football quarterback throws a pass, he aims it at a particular receiver. He doesn't just throw the ball in the air and hope someone will catch it. Likewise, the Basic Recipe needs to be aimed at a specific problem. Otherwise, it will bounce around aimlessly with little or no effect.

You "aim" the Basic Recipe by applying it while "tuned in" to the problem from which you want relief. This tells your system which problem needs to be the receiver.

Remember the discovery statement which states:

> *The cause of all negative emotions is a disruption in the body's energy system.*

Negative emotions come about because you are tuned into certain thoughts or circumstances which, in turn, cause your energy system to disrupt. Otherwise, you function normally. One's fear of heights is not present, for example, while one is reading the comic section of the Sunday newspaper and therefore not tuned in to the problem.

Tuning in to a problem can be done by simply thinking about it. In fact, tuning in *means* thinking about it. Thinking about the problem will bring about the energy disruptions involved which then...and only then...can be balanced by applying the Basic Recipe. Without tuning in to the problem…thereby creating those energy disruptions…the Basic Recipe does nothing.

Tuning in is seemingly a very simple process. You merely think about the problem while applying the Basic Recipe. That's it…at least in theory.

However, you may find it a bit difficult to consciously think about the problem while you are tapping, humming, counting, etc. That's why I'm introducing a Reminder Phrase that you can repeat continually while you are performing the Basic Recipe.

The Reminder Phrase is simply a word or short phrase that describes the problem and that you repeat out loud each time you tap one of the points in The Sequence. In this way you continually "remind" your system about the problem you are working on.

The best Reminder Phrase to use is usually identical to what you choose for the affirmation you use in the Setup. For example, if you are working on a fear of public speaking, the Setup affirmation would go like this…

Even though I have this <u>fear of public speaking</u>, I deeply and completely accept myself.

Within this affirmation, the underlined words…<u>*fear of public speaking*</u>…are ideal candidates for use as the Reminder Phrase.

I sometimes use a shorter version of this Reminder Phrase when in seminars such as those presented on our DVDs. I might, for example, use "public speaking fear" or just "public speaking" instead of the somewhat longer version shown above. That's just one of the shortcuts we have grown accustomed to after years of experience with these techniques. For your purposes, however, you can simplify your life by just using the identical words for the Reminder Phrase as you use for the affirmation in the Setup. That way you will minimize any possibility for error.

Now here's an interesting point that you will most certainly notice on the audios and some of the videos. *I don't always have people repeat a Reminder Phrase.* That's because I have discovered over time that simply stating the affirmation during the Setup is usually sufficient to "tune in" to the problem at hand. The subconscious mind usually locks on to the problem throughout the Basic Recipe even though all the tapping, humming, counting, etc. would seem to be distracting.

But this is not *always* true and, with extensive training and experience, one can recognize whether or not using the Reminder Phrase is necessary. As stated, it is not usually necessary but…*when it is necessary it is really necessary and must be used.*

What's beautiful about EFT is that you don't need to have my experience in this regard. You don't have to be able to figure out whether or not the Reminder Phrase is necessary. You can just *assume* it is always necessary and thereby assure yourself of always being tuned in to the problem by simply repeating the Reminder Phrase as instructed. It does no harm to repeat the Reminder Phrase when it is not necessary, and it will serve as an invaluable tool when it is. This is part of the 100-percent overhaul concept mentioned earlier. We do many things in each round of the Basic Recipe that may not be necessary for a given problem. But when a particular part of the Basic Recipe *is* necessary...*it is absolutely critical.*

It does no harm to include everything...even what may be unnecessary...and *it only takes one minute per round.* This includes *always* repeating the Reminder Phrase each time you tap a point during The Sequence. It costs nothing to include it...not even time...because it can be repeated within the same time it takes to tap each energy point seven times.

This concept about the Reminder Phrase is an easy one. But just to be complete, I am including a few samples below:

headache	*anger towards my father*
war memory	*stiffness in my neck*
nightmares	*craving for alcohol*
fear of snakes	*depression*

Subsequent Round Adjustments

Let's say you are using the Basic Recipe for some problem (fear, headache, anger, etc.). Sometimes the problem will simply vanish after just one round while, at other times, one round provides only partial relief. When only partial relief is obtained, you will need to do one or more additional rounds.

Those subsequent rounds need to be adjusted slightly for best results. Here's why: One of the main reasons why the first round doesn't always completely eliminate a problem is because of the re-emergence of Psychological Reversal...that interfering blockage that the Setup is designed to correct.

This time, Psychological Reversal shows up in a somewhat different form. Instead of blocking your progress altogether it now blocks any *remaining* progress. You have already made some headway but become stopped part way toward complete relief because Psychological Reversal enters in a manner that keeps you from *getting any better still.*

Since the subconscious mind tends to be very literal, the subsequent rounds of the Basic Recipe need to address the fact that you are working on the *remaining problem*. Accordingly, the affirmation contained within the Setup needs to be adjusted as does the Reminder Phrase.

Here's the adjusted format for the Setup affirmation:

Even though I still have some of this _____, I deeply and completely accept myself.

Please note the emphasized words (*still* and *some*) and how they change the thrust of the affirmation toward the *remainder* of the problem. It should be easy to make this adjustment and, after a little experience, you will fall into it quite naturally.

Study the adjusted affirmations below. They reflect adjustments to the original affirmations shown earlier in this section.

Even though I still have some of this fear of public speaking, I deeply and completely accept myself.

Even though I still have some of this headache, I deeply and completely accept myself.

Even though I still have some of this anger towards my father, I deeply and completely accept myself.

Even though I still have some of this war memory, I deeply and completely accept myself.

Even though I still have some of this stiffness in my neck, I deeply and completely accept myself.

Even though I still have some of these nightmares, I deeply and completely accept myself.

Even though I still have some of this craving for alcohol, I deeply and completely accept myself.

Even though I still have some of this fear of snakes, I deeply and completely accept myself.

Even though I still have some of this depression, I deeply and completely accept myself.

The Reminder Phrase is also easily adjusted. Just put the word *remaining* before the previously used phrase. Here, as examples, are adjusted versions of the previous Reminder Phrases.

remaining *headache*

remaining *anger towards my father*

remaining *war memory*

remaining *stiffness in my neck*

remaining *nightmares*

remaining *craving for alcohol*

remaining *fear of snakes*

remaining *depression*

If your pain disappears but then returns, simply repeat EFT's Basic Recipe and the "remaining pain" Reminder Phrase described above.

2

Optional Points
and Refinements

As EFT spread to those with a knowledge of acupuncture, many students and practitioners began to add tapping points. There are hundreds of acupuncture points on the human body—in fact, it's just about impossible to tap yourself anywhere without hitting one or more of them—but the most popular optional points in EFT circles are probably the top of the head and points on the wrists and ankles. None of these points are mentioned in the EFT Manual. Feel free to experiment with any or all of them.

Top of Head. Run an imaginary string over your head from the top of one ear to the top of the other. The highest point that the string reaches is the Top of Head point.

Wrists. Several meridians run through the inside and outside of the wrist. An easy way to stimulate all of the wrist points is to cross your wrists and tap them together (about where your wristwatch would be), inside wrist against inside wrist, inside wrist against outside wrist, and outside wrist against outside wrist.

Ankle Points. Several meridians run through the ankles. These are less widely used because they're less convenient, but many EFTers include them from time to time. To stimulate these points, simply tap on all sides of the ankle, using either or both legs.

In the reports shared by EFT users in this book and at theEFT website, you'll see other points mentioned, including some that are used in combination. I don't personally use those points or combinations so I won't elaborate on them here. EFT is so flexible and versatile that I am never surprised when any acupressure tapping combined with focused thought produces good results.

Possible Outcomes

There are five possible outcomes after a full round of EFT.

1. The pain level improves or goes away completely.

2. The location of the pain moves to another part of the body, even if it only moves an inch or two.

3. The quality of the pain changes from, let's say, a sharp pain to a dull ache, or from a throb to a tingle …and so on.

4. The pain level increases.

5. Nothing happens.

I'll cover what to do about each of these possibilities in detail, but please note that…

All of the changes in items 1 through 4 are evidence that EFT is working for you.

1. **What do I do if the pain level improves or goes away completely?** If the pain improves but doesn't go to zero, do more EFT rounds until it reaches zero or plateaus at some improved level. If it plateaus and three or four more EFT rounds don't result in relief then you can assume that "nothing more will happen" and go to item 5 below.

   If the pain goes away completely, you are done. You're one of our well-known "One-Minute Wonders," and while you may find it surprising, this is a frequent occurrence. Enjoy the results and get on with your life.

   If the pain disappears but resurfaces at another time, this is evidence that more EFT is necessary. It would be a mistake to conclude that EFT "didn't work" because it obviously did. Our bodies give us many valuable messages (if we are listening) and sometimes a single pain can have several causes. You can try more rounds of standard EFT on the pain and, eventually, the pain may subside permanently. If not, just assume that "nothing more will happen" and go to item 5 below.

2. **What do I do if the location of the pain moves to another part of the body, even if it only moves an inch or two?** Any movement of the pain is cause for optimism because it suggests that the original

pain has been alleviated in favor of another pain that now gets your attention. It could also mean that the original pain had an emotional cause that was "alleviated in the background" and the new pain is evidence of a new emotional cause. In either case, start over with EFT at the new location just as though it is a brand new pain—because it is.

If the pain moves again, then keep "chasing the pain" until the pain level falls to zero. If you get stuck on a pain that doesn't move or if you don't get relief after three or four diligent rounds of EFT, then assume that "nothing more will happen" and proceed to item 5 below.

3. **What do I do if the quality of the pain changes from, let's say, a sharp pain to a dull ache, or from a throb to a tingle...and so on?** This is similar to item 2 above except the pain changes nature or quality instead of location. Any such quality change is cause for optimism because it suggests that the original pain has been altered. In this case, start over with EFT as though this altered version is a new pain. Keep doing EFT rounds on any future altered pains until the pain level falls to zero. If you get stuck on an altered pain that doesn't move or if you don't get relief on it after three or four diligent rounds of EFT, then assume that "nothing more will happen" and proceed to item 5 below.

4. **What do I do if the pain level increases?** Although it doesn't happen often, I have certainly seen cases where pain levels increased after one or two rounds

of EFT. Many healing responses triggered by other therapies show signs of getting worse (they call it a "healing crisis") before getting better.

Three or four more rounds of EFT will usually "turn the corner" and launch noticeable relief. If not, or if the relief plateaus at a level above zero, then assume that "nothing more will happen" and proceed to item 5.

5. **What do I do if nothing happens?** The high likelihood here is that unresolved emotional issues are major contributors to the pain.

This may seem odd to you, especially if physicians have shown you X-rays or other physiological evidence explaining why you have pain. Nonetheless, I have lost count of the many "impossible pains" that have been relieved by applying EFT to anger, fear, trauma, and the like. As Dr. Sarno theorizes, the damaging chemicals and muscular tension caused by our negative emotions may be the largest contributor to pain.

It certainly appears that way to me. That's why this book should be so valuable to so many. It goes into areas where conventional medicine does not and that's why it often works where nothing else will.

So now we need to search for emotional causes to pain and apply EFT to them. Since we have so many differing emotional histories, this bit of detective work needs to be customized to you. I usually do this by asking questions. Here's one:

> *If there was a specific emotional event contributing to this pain, what could it be?*

The beautiful thing about this question is that it often points to a vital emotional cause even if it doesn't seem that way at first. Your system has a way of knowing what is going on even if you see no realistic link. For example, your back pain may seem to have no connection to the memory of your third grade teacher ridiculing you in front of the class. That's okay, just use EFT on that memory with a Setup Phrase like...

> *"Even though Mrs. Johnson humiliated me in third grade..."*

Do this for as many rounds as it takes to bring your current emotional intensity on this event down to zero. When completed, you are likely to notice relief from your pain. If not, ask the question again and use EFT on the resulting emotional issue. Repeated efforts at this are likely to have two benefits: the emotional events will have lost their sting (probably permanently), and your pain should have faded considerably.

Another good question is:

> *If you could live your life over again, what person or event would you just as soon skip?*

This question is more general than the previous one but its answer usually leads to important specific events that need collapsing. For example, if your answer to the above is "My brother Jake," then you can break down your experience with Jake into all the specific events you have had with him that left you feeling angry, frustrated, afraid, etc.

With these two questions, you can uncover and resolve important issues that limit your life and cause you pain and/or other symptoms. That's very useful.

One point, though. You *must* come up with an answer to these questions or they will be useless. A response like "I don't know" is unacceptable. If you really *don't* know, use the first guess that comes to mind. If you don't even have a guess, then *make one up!*

Often a made-up issue is as good as or better than a real one. That's because it still came from you and thus it isn't totally fictitious. It still has your experiences and emotions embedded within it and it can even blend several "forgotten issues" together in a useful way.

Touch and Breathe (TAB) Method

Not everyone enjoys or can do the vigorous, lively tapping that most EFTers employ, and in some situations—such as during a business meeting or when dining in public—tapping just doesn't feel comfortable for most people.

An effective alternative is the Touch and Breathe, or TAB, method developed by John Diepold, PhD. Instead of tapping on each acupoint, simply hold it with a fingertip while breathing in and breathing out. Start by holding your Sore Spot or Karate Chop point, or hold your hands together with Karate Chop points touching, while saying your Setup Phrase out loud or to yourself. Then touch and hold each of the EFT acupoints while taking a full breath in and out.

The Sequence takes a bit longer this way, but it can be more comfortable and relaxing, and it works. It's also less conspicuous. Some EFTers gently massage the acupoints, which is something many of us do instinctively while thinking or concentrating. They rub or press the upper lip, touch the Under Arm point while hugging themselves, stroke the collarbone, or scratch the top of the head.

To stimulate the hand points, hold each finger between the thumb and forefinger of the "tapping" hand while breathing in and breathing out, or place your fingertips together (index fingers touching, thumbs touching, etc.) and breathe. To activate the wrist points, simply circle your wrist with the opposite hand and hold it while breathing. To access the ankle points, reach down and touch the ankles while breathing.

One-minute Wonders

We use the term "one-minute wonder" to describe EFT sessions that produce immediate results, often in people who are trying it for the first time. In those situations, EFT can seem like magic. Sometimes the response is so immediate that there isn't time to complete the Basic Recipe or even an entire tapping sequence.

Here's an example from Jane Beard, who introduced someone to EFT at a dinner party with dramatic results in less than a minute.

Year-long Nagging Back Pain Gone in 30 Seconds

by Jane Beard

I was at a dinner party with many people I hadn't seen in a while, trying to explain what I am up to now, like studying EFT, and why.

One of them mentioned she had had a nagging pain in her back for most of this year. We measured her level of intensity and tapped on the Karate Chop point while she twice repeated the Setup Phrase, *"Even though I have this nagging pain in my lower back..."*

The third time we spoke the Setup, I added *"...and I'm willing to let this go."* Bingo! The pain left her body as she said the words. We did one round of tapping on the face and torso points and the top of the head (which I have come to call the "yarmulke spot") just for good measure. She was stunned, and so was everyone who saw it happen. Two days later, she was still pain free. That was 14 months ago, and this woman has been completely free from pain the entire time. It never came back.

❉ ❉ ❉

Here's another case in which the results, although they took longer than a minute, are nonetheless fast and remarkable. The pain, which had lasted for five years, disappeared in a few minutes thanks to basic EFT. Note how the author, Sylvia Ross, touches a pain spot before tapping. This helps the client "tune into" the specific pain.

Basic EFT Alleviates Long-term Back Pain

by Silvia Ross

I met with Bonnie, a 58-year-old neighbor, who had been diagnosed with Chronic Fatigue Syndrome (CFS) and fibromyalgia ten years ago. One morning she couldn't get out of bed and could barely move. She has a history of seizures but had not had any this past year. She is on six different medications, including a type of morphine for pain.

She had not had the opportunity to view the Introductory EFT video before her appointment, so that was the first step. The video is great—it makes believers out of first-time clients. Bonnie then gave me an overview of her history, which included mental and physical abuse from her mother, being a workaholic and perfectionist, and the list goes on.

As she told her story, her stress level was rising. I was concerned about her history of seizures so I had her stop and fill out a short intake form listing two symptoms with their levels of intensity on a scale of 0-to-10. The first was upper back pain with a level of intensity of 7 out of 10. The second was lower back pain with a level of intensity of 10 out of 10. She had had pain on and off for five years. She listed her basic wellbeing at a stress level of 6.

We did one round of EFT for pain in her back and I had her gently touch and tap all the points while I rubbed the Gamut Point on her right hand. It was all very soft-spoken as I was concerned about her seizure history, and the Setup statements were basic.

Even though I have this pain in my back at this intensity and all these memories have added to it, I completely love, accept, and forgive myself, and anyone else.

I asked for a rating on her pain, fully expecting not much movement, but after a look of puzzlement, she said, "It's gone!" Then she yawned at least ten times. I thought she might fall asleep at the table. At that point it was time for her to go. She talked about how wonderful she felt and said she wanted me to see her son, who has multiple sclerosis, and her husband, who also has back problems. Taking an EFT Chart, she promised to tap at home.

A couple of days later I stopped in to see how she was doing and again she told me how well she felt and her back pain had not returned. The only tapping I did with her that time was for a trigger point on the bottom of her foot which had hurt since she had major surgery on her ankle after a car accident. I touched the spot to make sure we had located it and then we did one simple round of EFT. Again the pain was gone!

For some reason, my touching the painful area before I do a round of tapping seems to benefit the process. I use it often and have had extremely good results. Usually one or two rounds will clear the pain. It seems to work even better than verbally describing the location in the Setup Phrase, which I also do.

Two Month Update: Bonnie's back pain has not returned! I saw her casually in her yard recently and she actually looked surprised when I asked her about her pain. She had gall bladder surgery a couple of weeks following her original session and had some complications from the surgery, but she assured me that she had no back pain.

✽ ✽ ✽

The Acceptance Phrase

The first element of every EFT Setup Phrase is a statement about the problem. But just as important is the second part, which is the Acceptance Phrase. The combined statement says that even though I have this problem, I accept myself. The Acceptance Phrase is an affirmation, which I consider crucial to the effectiveness of EFT.

But for many EFT students, the Setup Phrase is a stumbling block. In a typical workshop of several hundred people, as many as half feel uncomfortable saying, "I fully and completely accept myself." For some the incongruity is so severe that they literally can't speak.

EFT can help anyone resolve old emotional issues that contribute to low self-esteem or feelings of guilt or shame, but for now, if the Setup Phrase is a problem, try saying one of the following statements while you tap:

Even though I can't yet fully and completely accept myself, I would like to some day fully and completely accept myself.

Even though I can't quite fully and completely accept myself, I'll be okay.

Even though it's hard for me to say that I fully and completely accept myself, I can let go of my fear and do this work.

Even though I can't yet accept myself, I can and do acknowledge myself.

If it's still difficult to say that you fully and completely accept yourself, or if it feels untrue, try changing the Setup Phrase altogether to something like:

Even though I have this back pain, I would like to feel better.

Even though I have this back pain, I can enjoy life.

Even though I have this back pain, it's going away.

As you experiment with Setup Phrases, try different variations. For example, try saying,

Even though I have this back pain, I absolutely do accept myself.

Even though I have this back pain, I love and forgive myself.

Even though I have this back pain, I forgive and accept myself and I forgive anyone and anything that contributed in any way to this pain.

Setup Phrases, by the way, can be of any length. While tapping on the Karate Chop point or massaging the Sore Spot, say whatever you like about the problem. You can also talk *to* the problem. Your Setup Phrase can last for five or ten minutes or more. The more detailed, specific, colorful, and interesting your Setup Phrase, the more likely you are to experience good results. As you read examples of how people have treated back pain with EFT throughout this book, you'll begin to appreciate the important role that imagination and intuition play in this process. Be ready to let your own imagination and intuition work on your behalf as you start tapping.

Here are some recommendations by EFT practitioner Betty Moore-Hafter for softening the delivery of EFT's Acceptance Phrase. Her approach is ideal for those who need to tiptoe into their issues.

Soft Language to Ease the Acceptance Phrase
by Betty Moore-Hafter

As I understand it, the EFT Setup Phrase paves the way for healing by shifting the hard, locked-up energy of psychological reversal to the softer energy of self-acceptance. I have found that creative wording can be especially helpful toward this end. Here are some of my favorites:

1. "...with kindness and compassion" or "...without judgment"

These and similar words contribute an extra dimension of support and care, especially when the issue is a sensitive one. Tears often come to people's eyes as we add these simple words.

Even though I feel unworthy, I deeply and completely accept myself with kindness and compassion—it's been hard for me.

Even though I'm so afraid of rejection, I deeply accept myself with gentleness and compassion—I've been hurt a lot.

Even though I feel guilty for that mistake I made, I totally accept myself without judgment. I'm only human.

It was my friend and EFT colleague Carolyn Lewis who first suggested some of these expressions to me. We trade sessions and, being on the receiving end, I experienced first-hand how good it felt to hear these kind words—and how much emotion they brought up. For me, they went right to the heart. I highly recommend that fellow EFTers trade sessions. You can learn so much by being guided and sharing ideas.

2. "I want to bring healing to this."

Some people balk at the words, "I deeply accept myself" and say, "But I don't accept myself! I hate myself for this." One gentle way to proceed is to say:

Even though I don't accept myself, I can accept that this is just where I am right now. And even though I don't accept myself, I want to bring healing to this. I would like to feel better, find more peace, and reach more self-acceptance.

Whenever self-acceptance is difficult, just stating the intent for healing breaks the deadlock of self-rejection. Most people do want to heal and feel better.

3. "The truth is…"

These words can usher in powerful reframes. And when you reframe a situation while tapping, it does shift the energy and things begin to change.

Even though I crave this cigarette, the truth is, cigarettes are making me sick.

Even though I still feel guilty, the truth is, I've done nothing wrong. This is false guilt.

Even though I still feel responsible for my sister, the truth is, she is an adult. She's responsible for herself now.

4. "I'm willing to see it differently…"

Sometimes amazing things happen after adding the words, 'I'm willing to see it differently." One of my clients was convinced that she could never have a child because she might abandon that child the way her father abandoned her. As we tapped through her pain from the father issue, I began adding the phrase, "and I'm willing to see it differently."

Even though my father really hurt me, I love and accept myself, and I'm willing to see it differently.

After several rounds of tapping, she seemed calm and said thoughtfully, "You know, I think my father really did love me in his own way. That's all he was capable of." She felt at peace with it for the first time. And, when I heard from her later, she and her husband were talking about having children. She knew she was not her father and would do it differently. She saw it all differently.

I often tap the EFT points with alternating Reminder Phrases, such as: Beginning of eyebrow, "Still feel guilty." Side of eye, "But the truth is…" and so on.

5. "That was then and this is now."

When childhood pain is being healed, people often feel great relief when words like these are added.

Even though when I was eight years old, I cried alone and no one came. I deeply love and accept my young self. And that was then and this is now. Now I have lots of help and support.

Even though I still feel anxious, afraid that something bad will happen. I deeply accept myself. And even though my child self felt anxious all the time, afraid my father would explode, I love and accept that child self. That was then and this is now. Now I'm safe. I don't need this hyper-vigilance anymore. I can relax now.

6. "I'm open to the possibility…"

"Choice" statements (dscribed on page 133), are of course very empowering when we are ready for them. But sometimes stating a choice is too much of a stretch. Often, the gentlest way to introduce a better choice is to simply bring in the idea of possibility.

Even though I'm full of doubt that I can lose weight, I deeply accept myself and I'm open to the possibility that it may be easier than I think.

Even though I'm stuck in this anger and don't want to let it go, I'm open to the possibility that it would be nice to feel more peaceful about this.

Even though I don't think EFT will work for me, I deeply accept myself and I'm willing to entertain the possibility that maybe EFT will help. I'm ready for some help.

I believe that when we open the door of possibility just a crack, it is enough to start the healing process into motion.

With all of these phrases, you can keep "I deeply and completely accept myself" and add the extra phrase, or you can substitute the phrase. Experiment and see what works for you!

❂ ❂ ❂

3

Tap While You...

Those who are new to EFT often ask when and how frequently they should practice tapping. The answer is: As often as you like—or, better yet, as often as possible. EFT is very flexible and forgiving. The more often you practice, the sooner EFT becomes a familiar tool that you can use without effort. The more you use it, the better it works. The more you use it, the more likely you are to remember to use it when you really need it.

I usually recommend that you start by tapping

as soon as you wake up in the morning,

before every meal,

and before falling asleep at night.

That's five times a day right there. Tap whenever you use the bathroom or take a shower and you'll add a few more. Some EFTers tap whenever they come to a stop sign or red light. Quite a few tap while they walk. You don't have to do the entire Basic Recipe—just a few quick taps as time permits will help keep your energy balanced —and as soon as you have enough time, follow up with the complete sequence. Many EFTers tap before, during, or after they pray or meditate. It's no exaggeration to say that EFT tapping can improve any project or activity.

One of our EFT success stories is Irene Mitchell, whose leg was so badly shattered in a car accident that doctors did not expect her to live. When she survived, they warned her that she probably wouldn't walk again. She learned EFT while recuperating at a rehabilitation nursing home, and the first thing she used it for was pain relief. A few fast rounds of tapping would totally eliminate the pain in her leg and hip for as long as 90 minutes, and then she would tap again. In this way she was able to stop taking pain medication. She also used EFT to improve the results of her physical therapy sessions, in some cases accomplishing in ten minutes what most people need weeks to achieve. Thanks to EFT, Irene left the nursing home several months ahead of schedule and resumed her active life—which included parasailing on a cruise vacation and dancing onstage at Disneyland!

When asked how often she tapped, Irene answered, "At least a hundred times a day. EFT was my pain medication. It got me out of the wheelchair, and it helped me fix any problem that occurred. I encourage anyone who's reading this book to use EFT as often as possible. With EFT's help, your mind and emotions can be powerful allies in helping you live a pain-free life."

When you're in a hurry, try tapping on a single point, such as the Karate Chop point, while you focus on your pain or problem. If you watch our DVDs, you'll see a workshop in which the tapping worked perfectly, and it wasn't until we saw the video that anyone noticed that I had completely forgotten to include the EFT tapping points. All we did was tap on the Karate Chop point while reciting a Setup Phrase, and it worked.

If you get in the habit of tapping on the EFT acupoints without reciting a Setup Phrase or focusing your thoughts on anything specific, that alone will help keep your energy balanced and help you live a happier life. For example, try tapping to music. This is a popular activity in some EFT workshops—it keeps the group focused and energetic—and it's an easy way to avoid an energy slump in the afternoon. Teaching children to tap to music is a great way to introduce them to EFT. Tap at whatever rhythm feels right. Experiment with classical music, rock, ballads, opera, military marches, movie soundtracks, or whatever you most enjoy.

Tap while you read your email or work at the computer. Tap while you watch TV. Tap while you talk on the phone. Tap while you study—that's an easy way to improve your reading comprehension and recall. Tap right now as you read this page.

If you tap while you describe things that you've seen or experienced, your recollections are more likely to be accurate. In fact, EFT would probably significantly improve the accuracy of eye-witness testimony. In EFT, we use the Tell a Story and Watch a Movie techniques to help people describe difficult events without feeling emotionally overwhelmed. With their emotions under control, they are able to think, remember, and process information more efficiently. Several EFT practitioners have reported on tapping's incredible calming effect when applied immediately after an accident, tragedy, or disaster.

Here's a great tip from EFT practitioner Rick Wilkes, which appeared in our online newsletter. I think it has special application for those experiencing back pain because it deals with underlying issues easily and automatically, without conscious effort. Some have found that their back pain completely disappeared as a result of following Rick's simple instructions.

The Tap-While-You-Gripe Technique

by Rick Wilkes

Have you ever called a friend just to gripe about everything that's gone wrong in your day? The truth is that when things go wrong, we need to feel that we're not alone. So we turn to trusted friends and family to let off steam and be comforted. It's a natural part of being human. Most of us have been expressing our pain this way since we were very young children.

What I call "griping" is just a way to retell a story with emotional intensity. And there is scientific proof that this can help us. Recent brain studies show that there's an *opportunity* when we relive an experience to have the stored emotions of that experience heal...or become even more intense. As we recall the story and feel the emotions in our body, our brain is making a decision—one that can go either way! Here's how it works.

Let's say the story that we're telling is one in which we feel alone and unsupported. If we tell that story to a friend who is loving, present, kind, and comforting, chances are that our primitive emotional brain will no longer feel alone and unsupported, right? In the process of telling the story, we heal the emotional intensity. That is the ideal outcome.

Yet, how often has it happened to you that in the process of telling and retelling an intense story, explaining about how you were "done wrong" by someone else, you find that after the second or third or fourth retelling that the pain is now more intense than it was right after it happened? That's the risk of sharing our painful experiences with others, whether they are talk professionals or not—unless you are using a technique that consistently allows you to eliminate and then harmonize the emotional intensity. And EFT is just such a technique.

That is why I suggest that you always tap while you gripe. Tap while you complain. Tap every time you tell a story that has negative emotional intensity. Pretty soon, you'll probably notice you have a lot less in your life to gripe about!

Here's how you can get started:

You've had a bad day. You want to feel that there's someone out there that understands you, that cares about you, that takes your side. So you pick up the phone, and you call your best friend. Start tapping...and tap continuously while you talk to her!

(Karate Chop) *Ring...Ring...Hello?*

(Top of Head) *Oh I'm so glad I reached you.*

(Inside Eyebrow) *I have had such a terrible day!*

(Side of Eye) *I really need someone to talk to.*

(Under Eye) *Do you have a few minutes?*

(Under Nose) *First off, this *&^%$ boss of mine...*

(then Chin, Collarbone, Under Arm, Karate Chop, and back to Top of Head, etc.)

The order of the points doesn't matter. The number of taps at each point doesn't matter. You can tap one point that feels good the whole call if you want. You can use the finger points. Just tap continuously while you talk. Don't stop!

Why would we do this? We talk to others to feel better, don't we? But there are two approaches to griping and complaining. The first is, alas, the more common. It is to gather people to our side in the upcoming war. We tell a story to make us "right" and the other party "wrong." With this plan, we must *build* intensity in ourselves and in others while we plan revenge (or a lawsuit, divorce, or other dramatic action designed so we *win* and the other *loses*).

The other approach is to want to *heal* from an emotional pain, and we're mature enough to know that intensifying the fear by making us the "Victims" and others into the "Powerful Forces of True Evil" just creates war inside us, not peace.

We can make our healing far more likely if we just tap the acupoints while we express our hurt and our anger and our sadness and our feelings of being out of control. We use what has been human nature since cave folks sat around the fire—the need to tell our story to tribe members to gain their supportive energy—and we use that supportive energy in a new way that is far more likely to result in a sense of peace for all of us.

What I find is that tapping while I gripe and complain shifts my entire perspective. As the noise of the emotional disruption settles down, I am far more likely to hear my intuition guide me to steps that resolve the situation in the best possible way.

Try it for yourself. Tap the acupoints while you are on the phone. No one needs to know that you are tapping. And just notice whether you see a change that helps you feel both more peaceful and more empowered. I am confident you will.

In fact, you may find this so effective that you pick up your phone and tap while you gripe without even calling your friend. Once you get it all out of your system, then you dial...and perhaps have a very different kind of conversation.

✳ ✳ ✳

Can You Do EFT Incorrectly?

This is an interesting question. EFT is so forgiving and versatile that finding ways in which it doesn't work can be a challenge. In fact, many EFTers respond that the only way to do it wrong is to not use it.

You *can* do an incomplete EFT treatment (which will make more sense as we explore core issues and other advanced concepts), but if you combine focused thought and intention with tapping, your efforts will probably work no matter what Setup Phrase or modified Tapping Sequence you use.

For example, you can omit the words "Even though" and simply state the problem:

My back hurts.

You can omit the "I completely and fully accept myself" phrase and simply say:

I'm okay.

This, by the way, is how we use EFT with children. A child who's upset can say:

Even though I flunked the math test, I'm a cool kid, I'm okay.

Even though I lost my backpack and I'm mad at myself, I'm still an awesome kid.

And you don't have to tap on the EFT acupoints in any specific order. I recommend the Sequence described here because it's easy to remember, but you can:

tap from top to bottom

tap from bottom to top

tap on every other point, then tap on the remaining points

tap first on one side of the body, then the other

tap on one side of the body and not the other

tap really fast, at a rate of several taps per second

tap really fast, moving at record speed from one point to the next

tap very slowly, at the rate of one tap or less per second

tap very slowly, staying for a full minute or more at each point

tap on a single point and forget about the rest

tap on a photo or drawing of yourself, another person, or an animal

tap mentally, in your head, without touching the points at all

And the list goes on. I believe that if your intention is to treat a specific issue, like the pain in your lower back, and you combine that intention with any type of acupoint stimulation, you can expect good results.

When I created EFT, I streamlined more complicated meridian therapies that involved separate algorithms or tapping patterns for different conditions or symptoms. Each had its own sequence. An algorithm for chronic pain, for example, started at the Inside Eyebrow point and went to Side of Eye, Under Eye, Under Nose,

Collarbone, Under Arm, Little Finger, Collarbone, Index Finger, and Collarbone, then ended with 50 taps on the Gamut point. An algorithm for anger, bitterness, and resentment moved from Inside Eyebrow to Little Finger to Collarbone. An algorithm for emotional trauma went from the Inside Eyebrow to Side of Eye, Under Eye, Under Arm, Collarbone, Thumb, Under Arm, Collarbone, Little Finger, Collarbone, and Index Finger.

I realized that these algorithms, which are difficult to remember, especially in emergencies, could be replaced with a single tapping pattern. By the time you complete three or more rounds of tapping on the EFT acupoints, you've tapped on all of the points in a variety of combinations. The beauty of meridian therapies is that when you stimulate points that you don't need, you don't hurt yourself or cause complications—and when you tap on points that you do need, the process works.

At first I replaced algorithms with a single tapping sequence and created EFT's Basic Recipe. Then I put the 9 Gamut treatment on the shelf, for use only when I'm stuck. Then I did the same with the finger points. These tools are worth learning because they can be very helpful, but if you get good results without them, why use them? Save them for when you need them.

I now encourage people to find their own "personal" EFT acupoint and try it first. Most of us, if we pay attention, realize that we're drawn to a certain point, or we notice that every time our energy shifts, it's when we're tapping on the same point. For some it's the Under Eye; for many, it's the Under Arm or Karate Chop point. For me, it's the Collarbone point. If you set out to relieve your back pain and you tap on a single acupoint and the pain goes away, you're done. What could be simpler?

Those who work only with mechanical EFT get good results most of the time. But mechanical EFT is not the only way, or even the official way, to use this technique. It's the foundation of EFT, and as soon as you start building on that foundation by experimenting, trying new approaches, and exploring new ways of presenting and using EFT, the sooner you will enjoy the exciting and often amazing results that this versatile procedure provides.

How to Tell Whether EFT Is Working

Did your tapping make a difference? When the problem is pain, the test is simple—either the pain goes away or it doesn't. If it does, it's probably because EFT successfully removed energy blocks while neutralizing emotional issues that were the pain's underlying cause. But pain relief isn't the only indication of EFT's effectiveness. Here are some common signs of EFT at work in any tapping session.

- *The person sighs*. This often happens after a round of tapping and it reflects an energy shift away from stress toward relaxation.

- *The person yawns*. The yawn might or might not be accompanied by fatigue. Some people have fallen asleep in the middle of their EFT sessions, but even well-rested people yawn during and after tapping.

Yawning has been associated with sleepiness, boredom, and (incorrectly) low blood oxygen levels. Behaviorists consider yawning a calming signal, a non-threatening bit of body language designed to help those nearby relax and feel safe. Recent research suggests that yawning is a way to cool the brain. Whatever its purpose, yawning in an EFT session is an important clue that energy is moving and the tapping is working.

- *The person's breathing changes.* Most of us breathe shallowly, especially when we're under stress. Longer, slower, deeper breaths are almost always a signal that EFT is working. The more balanced your energy, the smoother and more relaxed your breathing.

- *The person's voice changes.* During an EFT session it's not uncommon for someone's voice to crack, for stress or tension to make the voice actually squeak, or for the person to have trouble talking. Then, after EFT brings the person's energy into balance, his or her voice sounds deeper, rounder, fuller, more confident, stronger, and more vibrant. Speech patterns change, too, going from stumbling and inarticulate to clear, coherent, fluid, and eloquent.

- *The person's posture and body language change.* People who are depressed, anxious, frightened, or in pain sit, stand, and walk very differently from the way they do when they're comfortable, confident, relaxed, happy, and healthy. In successful EFT sessions, postural changes are often obvious. Instead of sitting hunched, with the head down and a curved spine, most people straighten up, lift their heads, and look at the world around them. Some practitioners describe their clients as blossoming like flowers as their energy clears.

- *The person cries.* The Tearless Trauma Technique is at the heart of EFT, and it really is possible to work through serious problems without weeping. But in many cases people do cry. Tears are often a sign of release or relief. Even if the tears are a symptom of discomfort, in which case the Tearless Trauma Technique is used to reduce the discomfort level, the emotional change indicates that EFT is working.

- *Sinuses drain.* Congested sinuses that suddenly begin to drain reflect an energy shift.

- *Facial muscles relax.* Actually, muscles all over the body soften, but changes in facial expression, such as from tense and stressed to relaxed and comfortable, are obvious clues. EFT can make such a difference in facial expression that some practitioners call it an instant face-lift. A few rounds of effective tapping can help you look years younger as well as happier.

- *Blood pressure and pulse change.* Often people begin an EFT session with an elevated pulse rate or high blood pressure. In those cases, successful EFT tapping—even if it's for something unrelated to physical symptoms—brings both pulse and blood pressure back to normal.

- *The person feels hot or cold.* A temperature change, such as feeling suddenly hot or cold, is another indication that EFT is working. A small or large area of back pain may feel intensely warm or hot, and the pain may pulse or vibrate. Someone who feels suddenly hot may blush or turn red. Another person might break out in a cold sweat and suddenly feel chilled. All of these physiological changes indicate that EFT is working.

- *The person feels vibrating energy.* Do enough tapping and your fingers will begin to tingle. When that happens, move your open hands toward each other, moving them closer, further apart, and closer again. If you sense a vibrating energy field or a feeling of resistance that grows stronger as your hands move closer, something is happening energetically.

- *A cognitive shift occurs.* One minute you're angry and the next you're laughing. One minute the person you're mad at can't do anything right and the next you're making excuses for him. One minute you're convinced that there is only one way, one "right" and "true" way, to look at the situation and the next you realize there are many. As soon as you stop replaying a situation in the same old way and notice something new or different, and as soon as "the principle of the thing" no longer matters the way it did, it's obvious that EFT has done its job.

- *The pain moves.* This happens so often that we use the phrase "chasing the pain" to describe the appropriate EFT response. The pain might move a short distance, such as an inch or two, but it's often a longer distance, such as from the left eye to the right side of the forehead or from the right shoulder blade to the center of the spine. In some cases pain jumps all over the body. For example, you might be tapping for pain in the small of your back and suddenly realize that your back pain has disappeared but now your right ankle is throbbing. Moving pain is a definite indication that EFT is working.

- *The pain gets worse*. Ironically, this can be a sign that EFT is working. It often indicates that buried emotional issues are getting close to the surface. By continuing to tap and by approaching the pain and its aspects from a different perspective, your results will probably improve. It's very unusual for pain to get worse and stay worse when you're using EFT, especially when you incorporate the many shortcuts and advanced techniques explained in this book.

- *The person is suddenly open to new options.* This is an excellent sign because it shows that the person is no longer stuck in his or her old way of thinking and feeling. Balanced energy leads to clear thinking.

You could say that the overall test is whether *any* kind of change is taking place. The more things change, the more energy is moving and the more EFT is working. Even if you haven't yet achieved the results you hope for, all this moving energy is a very good sign. It's only when nothing happens — the pain stays exactly where it was, the person's attitude doesn't shift at all, and the whole situation stays stuck — that we are tempted to conclude that EFT was not effective.

Even when that happens, it's worth trying again. So much depends on the art of delivery, the search for core issues, and the examination of different aspects that a sudden breakthrough can turn an unresponsive situation into an EFT success story. I've seen this so many times that I never conclude that EFT "didn't work." Rather, I adopt the belief that EFT always works but that sometimes we have to keep searching for the problem's true emotional cause.

The next chapter will help you develop the EFT skills that bring outstanding results for yourself and your own pain, for every other problem you'd like to solve, and for anyone else—including friends, relatives, co-workers, total strangers, and even family pets. In fact, our files include reports from people who used EFT to improve the health of their house plants and the performance of their cars, computers, and household appliances.

I shouldn't be surprised. After all, I told them to try it on everything! And you can, too.

4

Exploring Underlying Issues

Every once in a while, someone tries the basic EFT formula and gets immediate, lasting results. "One-Minute Wonders" can and do happen, even with incapacitating back pain.

But in many cases, at some point after mechanical EFT reduces or eliminates the pain, it comes back. If this happens to you, don't assume that EFT didn't work. EFT worked fine on the problem you treated, but now a new aspect has presented itself, and that aspect needs attention, too.

Introducing Aspects

Aspects are the various facets, features, portions, and pieces of a situation. Although EFT resolves many problems in a straightforward manner, different aspects can complicate just about any problem you address with EFT. Fortunately, they can be handled easily.

Consider all the aspects of back pain. In addition to having underlying emotional causes, which can be many, the pain you experience while lying down may be different from the pain you experience while standing up. The pain you experience while walking can be different from the pain you feel while bending or stretching. Other aspects include your location, companions, activities, surroundings, sights, sounds, smells, and experiences. The pain is probably linked to past events that are linked to other past events, creating a daisy chain of things that happened. The links that tie the events together exist only in your mind, but linked they are, from the present moment back to childhood.

Aspects are important in EFT. Each aspect qualifies as a separate problem even when they all relate to the same pain or the same larger problem. Some problems have so many pieces or aspects that the difficulty will not be completely resolved until all of them—or at least several of them—are addressed.

Experienced EFTers often compare this procedure to peeling an onion. You get rid of one layer only to discover another. When a problem has many layers or aspects, neutralizing them with EFT can seem like a daunting project. But considering how quickly those layers can be dealt with and how beneficial the results are, the project is more exciting than intimidating. And the rewards are priceless.

Be Specific

If you want fast, impressive results with EFT, be specific. Vague statements generate vague outcomes. The biggest mistake made by newcomers is using EFT on issues that are too global. Global problems are broad and hazy. They aren't well defined. Even with perseverance, which can almost always make a difference, global statements are less likely to produce results than specific statements about specific events.

I have been beating the drum for many years about being specific with EFT, urging EFTers to break emotional issues into the events that underlie them. When we do this, we address true causes and not just symptoms. While there is a skill to doing this, those who take this approach have watched their success rates climb impressively. They are also doing deeper, more meaningful work.

I have found, and demonstrated consistently, that applying EFT to the *smallest component* of a bothersome memory almost always works. In fact, I have rarely failed to gain success in this way in my last several hundred attempts. This idea has the potential to substantially improve EFT's success rate and pave the way for healing in areas previously thought difficult or impossible.

Many newcomers to EFT present their emotional issues in very global terms. They say things like:

I feel abandoned.	*I'm always anxious.*
I was an abused child.	*I hate my father.*
I have low self-esteem.	*I can't do anything right.*
I'm depressed.	*I feel overwhelmed.*

To them, *that* is the problem and *that* is what they want EFT to fix.

But, despite the person's perception, *that* is not the problem at all. Those feelings are merely symptoms of the problem. The real problem is that unresolved specific events, memories, and emotions cause the larger issue. How can one feel abandoned or abused, for example, unless specific events occurred in one's life to cause those feelings? The feelings didn't just appear out of the ether. They must have had a cause.

If we consider the larger issue (such as abandonment) to be a table top, then the table's legs represent specific events that support the table (my mother died when I was seven; my father walked out on us when I was eleven; I got lost on a hiking trip in the Sierra mountains; etc.).

Obviously, if we reduce an issue to the specific events supporting it and then collapse its table legs, the table top will fall for lack of support. In this way we address the true causes (specific events and emotions linked to them) rather than just symptoms.

Unfortunately, many EFT practitioners still apply EFT to the table top and not the supporting table legs. Thus they might start with...

Even though I have this feeling of abandonment...

Being too global like this is the number-one error made by new EFTers and some seasoned ones, too. Interestingly, this approach will sometimes get results but it is not nearly as thorough or precise as going for the supporting table legs first.

Also, because this global approach lacks precision, those using it are more likely to report that their issues "come back." What "come back," of course, are unresolved aspects (table legs) that were not previously addressed.

In addition, approaching an issue in a vague or global manner creates an environment in which the person's attention shifts from event to event. You can be much more accurate and achieve greater success if you reduce those global issues (table tops) to the specific events (table legs) that cause them. Examples for the global issue of "I feel abandoned" could include:

The time my mother left me in the shopping mall when I was in second grade.

The time my father told me to leave home when I was twelve.

The time my third-grade teacher gave me that "I don't care about you" look.

These specific events are much easier to deal with than the global issues they created. If you deal with them one at a time without letting your attention shift, it will be easy to clear them—and by clearing the emotions stored in these small specific events, you'll automatically repair the larger global issue.

Defining the Pain

EFT practitioners like to ask questions, and for many newcomers, the questions are unusual or downright weird. But if you enter into the spirit of the game, specific questions, especially those that invite you to use your imagination, can remove some of the barriers that surround chronic pain and its underlying issues. To help improve your receptiveness to these ideas, tap on the EFT acupoints while you read and answer the following. The examples that follow are from actual EFT clients and students.

1.   **Describe the pain.** Where is it? How big is it? What shape is it? What number do you give it on the 0-to-10 scale?

> *It's a rectangular box about the size and shape of a videotape buried deep in my shoulder, and it's a 9 right now*

> *It's a flattened oval, the size and shape of a squashed grapefruit. It covers my lower back. I can't move. It's a 10.*

> *It's three small hard marbles in my upper right hip. When I press against them the pain is a 6 or 7. When I try to do yoga, it's a 9 or 10.*

> *It's a heavy wet blanket that covers my spine. It's a pretty constant 5 or 6. I can still walk and move, but it hurts all the time and weighs me down, and I always know it's there.*

2.   **What color is it?** Is it bright or dull? Glossy or matte? Solid or dappled? Vivid or muted? Neon or pastel? Transparent or opaque? Clear or hazy? Blurry or in focus?

> *It's bright yellow with orange flecks at the edges like a flame.*

> *It's a deep red-orange.*

> *It's navy blue, like a dark velvet blue.*

It's a bright, clearly delineated orange oval surrounded by an indistinct reddish swirling cloud.

It's a grimy dull mustard yellow. It needs a bath.

It's a bright electric neon blue.

It's black. When it lightens up, it's charcoal gray.

3. **What is its texture?** Is it rough or smooth? Hard or soft? Solid or spongy? Does it hold its shape or shift and change?

It's hard with a rough, grainy surface.

It's very hard and spiky, with thorns all over.

It's soft and oozy, like Jell-O. It undulates.

It's fuzzy.

It's raspy, like rough sandpaper.

It's a ball of electricity that shoots lightning bolts down my spine.

It's thin and sharp like a needle or an ice pick.

4. **Does it make a sound?** Do you hear a noise, a voice, a rustle, a crackle?

It's a dull, heavy, background roar, like highway traffic.

It crackles, like a wood fire or like paper burning.

It's shrill, like a dentist's drill.

I hear a lot of static.

It grates and grinds, making a noise like gravel.

5. **Is the pain steady, or does it pulse or throb?** Is the throbbing intermittent or ongoing? Does the pain come in waves? Does it have a rhythm?

It's a dull, throbbing, monotonous pain that never stops.

It comes and goes. When I least expect it, it zaps me hard.

It's like the tides. It starts in the morning at a low level and rises up all day, then at night it recedes.

It moves in ripples or waves, starting in my right hip and moving across my back to my left shoulder.

6. **What does the pain remind you of?** One way to get a good answer to this important question is to say, "This pain reminds me of ____," or, "This pain makes me think of ____," and wait for your mind to fill in the blank.

This pain reminds me of being sick when I was a kid and feeling totally helpless.

This reminds me of the time I painted the house because I couldn't afford to hire anyone and I sprained my back.

This pain makes me think of how much I hate my job.

This pain makes me think about my sister-in-law and all the time I had to spend with her planning my niece's wedding. I'm still exhausted.

7. **When did the pain first appear?** What were you doing? What was happening in your life? What is your pain's history?

This pain started the week my brother got arrested.

This pain started right after I found out I was pregnant.

The day I got laid off, I came home from work and tripped on the stair. I've been hurting ever since.

My back has been in spasms ever since my wife walked out on me.

8. **How does the pain make you feel?** This is another crucial question because EFT is Emotional Freedom Techniques, and emotions are the underlying cause of most pain. Does the pain make you angry, frustrated, upset, sad, depressed, irritated, or confused?

    I feel guilty because I'm impatient with everyone, including the cat.

    Are you kidding? I'm furious! This pain has wrecked my life!

    I get so discouraged. Everything's an effort. Nothing seems to help. Why bother trying?

    I'm worried about everything—my business, the kids, money. All I do is hurt and feel sick about not being able to do anything.

9. **Is there anything else we need to know about this pain?** A good way to ask this question is to say, "This pain must be here because _____," or, "This pain makes me realize _____."

    This dark gloomy black awful wet blanket of pain must be here because my adjustable rate mortgage is going up again, I may lose the house, and I'm too depressed to think straight.

    This bright orange ball of pain in my lower back makes me realize how much I hate living next door to my sister.

    This pain makes me realize what a big mistake it was to buy a new truck.

This pain is here to punish me for what I did last summer.

10. **Has your condition been diagnosed by a physician?**
    If so, including this information is another way to be specific. For many, a medical diagnosis complete with official terminology makes the diagnosis "real."

    Even though I was diagnosed with herniated nucleus pulposus lumbar spine at the L5 level...

    Even though I have a C5-C6 cervical herniated disc that is compressing my spinal cord...

    Even though I have degenerative adult scoliosis...

If you don't have a specific diagnosis, you can still take advantage of the power that medical terminology holds over most of us. Borrowing from the preceding descriptions of back pain, consider saying:

Even though I have deep, throbbing nociceptive pain resulting from old injuries and involving muscle tension, changes in circulation, postural imbalances, psychological distress, neurological effects, spontaneous excitation of the central nervous system, and changes in my limbic-hypothalamic system...

Even though I have chronic neuropathic pain from nerve damage, resulting in exaggerated responses to painful stimuli and constant or intermittent burning, aching, shooting, or stabbing pain that fires spontaneously at old injury sites and at other locations along the nerve pathway...

As you examine the pain, keep tapping and adding to your description so that your Setup Phrase keeps growing. Remember, the Setup Phrase can be as long as you like, and the more you talk to yourself about the pain, the more likely you are to create descriptions that work.

Even though I have this pain that's the size and shape of a squashed grapefruit in the small of my back...

Even though I have this bright orange grapefruit-sized pain in the small of my back...

Even though I have this hard, spiky, thorny bright orange pain the size of a squashed grapefruit in the small of my back...

Even though I have this hard, spiky, thorny bright orange pain the size of a squashed grapefruit that doesn't make any noise, it's quiet and lethal...

Even though I have this hard, thorny, silent spiky bright red-orange grapefruit pain that shoots flaming lightning bolts that stab like sharp needles through my lower back and up my spine...

This hard, thorny red-orange pain reminds me of when I had a tooth infection and had to go to the dentist, and I felt so helpless and frustrated....

Even though this spiky orange grapefruit pain is interfering with everything in my life so I can't do anything or go anywhere, I can't work, I can't think, it's so frustrating, it makes me so angry, I'm so upset, I feel so helpless, I'm just a wreck, and it's all because of this grapefruit in my back...

11. **When you finish tapping, test your results.** Can you move? Can you stand, sit, bend, walk, or whatever you couldn't do before? Compare your pain now to the pain you described at the beginning of this exercise. Measure it on the Intensity Scale. Picture its

size, shape, color, texture, and other descriptions. How is it different?

Now my hard red-orange spiky thorny grapefruit pain is a small square box. It isn't red-orange any more, it's lime green. It isn't spiky or thorny any more, it's smooth. It isn't a 10 any more on the pain scale, it's a zero. It isn't angry and disruptive any more, it's well behaved and apologetic. It didn't mean to hurt me. I feel safe now. I don't feel helpless. When I bend to the left or right, I can't find any pain at all.

It was dark brownish yellow and now it's very pale, clear, pastel yellow, almost transparent. It was the size and shape of a golf ball, and now it's smaller than a marble. It hurts a lot less, but I can still feel it when I stand up. I'd say it went from an 8 to a 2 or maybe a 3.

12. **Measure your progress.** If the pain has completely disappeared, congratulations! Enjoy resuming your normal activities. If the pain has improved but has not completely disappeared, start your next round of EFT with "Even though I still have…" That's the Setup Phrase to use for whatever pain may be left, for pain that has moved, and for pain that has changed its shape and size but is still with you.

Even though the pain is still there a little…

Even though I still have some of this pain in a small smooth navy blue box on the right side of my spine just below my neck…

Even though I still have some of this pain in a soft, round green grape that's stuck in my left shoulder… It's barely a

3 but it's still there, but I can feel it getting softer and dissolving...

The "Core Issues" of Back Pain

Core issues are the major events or problems that underlie our symptoms. When it comes to back pain, core issues are the gold nuggets that, if we can only find and treat them with EFT, provide rapid relief.

The problem with core issues is that they're not always easy to find. We hide them from ourselves. They're painful. Our subconscious minds don't want us to go there. Our conscious minds are usually clueless —they have no idea what events or memories are lurking beneath the surface or how those events and memories might be causing pain.

In his book *The Divided Mind*, John Sarno, MD, describes Tension Myositis Syndrome, or TMS, as a modern pain-causing epidemic. "In this condition," he writes, "the brain orders a reduction of blood flow to a specific part of the body, resulting in mild oxygen deprivation, which causes pain and other symptoms, depending on what tissues have been oxygen-deprived."

According to Dr. Sarno, in addition to afflicting millions with back pain, sore necks, painful joints, carpal tunnel syndrome, fibromyalgia, post-polio syndrome, and muscle strains, TMS is the underlying cause of digestive problems such as gastroesophageal reflux, peptic ulcer, hiatus hernia, irritable bowel syndrome, and spastic colitis, as well as tension headache, migraine headache, prostatitis, sexual dysfunction, and tinnitus (ringing in the ears). That's quite a list!

Where does pain come from and why? According to Dr. Sarno, pain serves only one purpose. He disagrees with those who believe that pain protects us from further injury or that it has other physiological benefits. Dr. Sarno believes that pain is a reaction to an unconscious emotion and that its sole purpose is to distract the mind from that emotion. He explains:

> Psychosomatic symptoms are created to assist the repression of rage and other unacceptable feelings. Although it is not entirely clear why these unconscious feelings strive to become conscious, it is abundantly clear why the brain resists the attempt. Some of those feelings are believed to be too dangerous or embarrassing or otherwise unacceptable to be brought into the light of day, while others are simply too painful to be experienced consciously.

To eliminate their pain, Dr. Sarno instructs his patients and readers to recognize pain as a symptom of anger and other negative emotions. He tells them to resume their normal lives instead of lying in bed or restricting their activities. He says that simply understanding the mind-body connection and realizing that their backs hurt because they are angry is enough to cure most patients.

Dr. Sarno is a professor of Rehabilitation Medicine at the New York University School of Medicine. It's startling to read a book in which a physician of his stature attacks the medical profession for misunderstanding the causes of back pain, routinely misdiagnosing this condition, and prescribing ineffective treatments that have nothing to do with pain's actual roots. He explains that patients are almost always misinformed and frightened by their medical and non-medical advisors, whose advice tends to worsen their back pain symptoms.

The four sources of rage that Dr. Sarno instructs his patients to watch for are

1. Harmful emotions, such as anger, hurt, and sadness, that can be traced back to childhood;

2. Anger stemming from self-imposed pressures to be perfect and good;

3. Anger generated by the pressures of life; and

4. Miscellaneous emotions like guilt, shame, insecurity, fear, and vulnerability, which also feed the anger reservoir.

His compelling theory leads straight to EFT, which can neutralize harmful emotions in record time, and to our search for core issues.

You could simply use mechanical EFT and say, "Even though my back hurts, I fully and completely accept myself," but if you want to address the pain so it goes away and never comes back, it's time to start delving beneath the surface by asking yourself the right questions. It's like being a detective.

Some questions that are routinely asked by EFT practitioners in this situation are:

When did the pain begin? What were you doing? What was going on in your life? Who was with you? What happened in your relationship? What was going on at work? Sometimes the answers are obvious. Sometimes they're not.

If you can't think of any obvious connections right away, let your mind relax and drift while you think, "If only…" All of us have "if only" moments. They're sad and filled with remorse or regret. *If only I had married Jane… If only I hadn't moved to Los Angeles… If only I'd stayed in school…*

"If I could do it all over" is a similar statement. What would you do over? What person or event would you skip if you could live your life again?

The Personal Peace Procedure

In my online tutorial, I describe the *Personal Peace Procedure,* which is an easy exercise that can be worked on whenever you practice EFT. Try it now. The sooner you start, the sooner you'll experience true personal peace.

1. **Make a list.** On a blank sheet of paper, make a list of every bothersome specific event you can remember. If you don't find at least 50, you are either going at this half-heartedly or you have been living on some other planet. Many people will find hundreds.

2. **List everything.** While making your list you may find that some events don't seem to cause you any current discomfort. That's okay. List them anyway. The mere fact that you remember them suggests a need for resolution.

3. **Give each event a title** as though it is a mini-movie. Examples: *Dad hit me in the kitchen — I stole Suzie's sandwich — I almost slipped and fell into the Grand Canyon — My third grade class ridiculed me when I gave that speech — Mom locked me in a closet for two days — Mrs. Adams told me I was stupid.*

4. **Tap for the big ones.** When the list is complete, pick out the biggest redwoods in your negative forest and apply EFT to each one of them until you either laugh about it or just can't think about it any more. Be sure to notice any aspects that may come up and consider them separate trees in your negative forest. Apply EFT to them accordingly. Be sure to keep after each event until it is resolved. After the biggest redwoods are removed, look for the next-biggest, etc.

5. **Work on at least one event movie per day** — preferably three — for three months. It takes only minutes per day. At this rate you will have resolved 90 to 270 specific events in three months. Then notice how your body feels better. Note, too, how your threshold for getting upset is much lower. Note how your relationships are better and how many of your therapy type issues just don't seem to be there any more. Revisit some of those specific events and notice how those previously intense incidents have faded into nothingness. Note any improvements in your blood pressure, pulse, and breathing ability, and of course note the improvements in your back pain and range of motion.

I ask you to consciously notice these things because, unless you do, the quality healing you will have undergone may be so subtle that you don't notice it. You may even dismiss it by saying, "Oh well, it was never much of a problem anyway." This happens repeatedly with EFT and thus I bring it to your awareness.

6. **If necessary, see your physician.** If you are taking prescription medications, you may feel the need to discontinue them. Please do so ONLY under the supervision of a qualified physician.

It is my hope that the Personal Peace Procedure will become a worldwide routine. A few minutes per day will make a monumental difference in school performance, relationships, health, and our quality of life. But these are meaningless words unless you put the idea into practice. As my good friend Howard Wight writes, "If you are ultimately going to do something important that will make a real difference…do it now."

The Watch a Movie and Tell a Story Techniques

In our search for core issues, we often use the Movie and Story Techniques. In both methods, you review a past event while tapping to reduce its emotional charge. The difference between the two is that in the Movie Technique, you watch events unfold in your mind, as though you're watching a movie, while in the Story Technique, you describe the events aloud.

The "plot" of the movie or story is usually very short. The key event lasted only a few seconds or a minute at most. However, if jumping straight to the key event is too painful, the movie or story can begin a few minutes before the key event.

The event may have hurt, but its retelling doesn't have to.

Unlike psychotherapy techniques that require clients to relive unpleasant past events in excruciating detail, EFT's approach is gentle and flexible. You watch the movie or tell the story until you reach a point that feels uncomfortable. Instead of forcing yourself to push on, step back and tap until the emotional intensity fades.

When you feel comfortable again, resume the movie or story. When feelings rise up again, take a step back and tap. In this simple two-steps-forward and one-step-back process, you can revisit any trauma and completely neutralize its emotional impact in minutes.

Our bodies store traumas, and our mental movies are keys that unlock emotions that are stored with those traumas. Because EFT tapping reduces the emotional charge attached to past events, it transforms the traumas, memories, energy blocks, targeted body parts, and emotions that were previously locked together. With the emotional charge gone, the traumas become normal memories, the connections disappear, and the pain once associated with them vanishes as well.

The Tearless Trauma Technique

The Movie and Story Techniques are powerful and effective, but in some situations, as gentle as they are, they can still be too intense, too overwhelming, too frightening, or too uncomfortable.

I always remind people that in EFT, you don't have to feel worse in order to feel better. If the memory of a traumatic past event is simply too painful to think about, the Tearless Trauma Technique can help.

Since I first introduced this technique, it has been used with great success by many. However, the term "tearless" does not mean that no one has ever shed tears or experienced discomfort while using it. Indeed, some people respond with tears or other forms of distress at the mere mention of their issue. Please consider the Tearless Trauma Technique as a method for eliminating distress with a minimum of discomfort.

In most of our EFT work, we recreate specific memories and then tap to neutralize their emotional charge. But in the Tearless Trauma Technique, we don't recreate anything. We just think about the traumatic event from a distance, in the most general way, while tapping.

I know that procedures that avoid or minimize emotional pain are criticized by some members of the healing community who believe that traumatic experiences must be thoroughly re-experienced before they can be completely relieved. I personally don't see why pain is at all necessary for healing to take place, although I would welcome debate on this. I feel confident saying this because I have taken care of a mountain of traumatic incidents (some of them *very* severe) and, after their healing, the clients have no interest at all in exploring insights or analyzing the "why" of their past experiences. More importantly, they are for the first time in their lives free from incapacitating emotional pain, and the results last. The pain never returns.

As soon as their energy shifts, there is a visible and obvious cognition change in the way these clients talk about once-troublesome incidents. They seem done with their issues because the resolution that is so highly valued by more intense techniques seems to take place within the EFT session with minimal pain. To me, this is so profound that it tempts me to rename the process "Peace without Pain."

The Tearless Trauma Technique works well in groups, in one-on-one sessions, and even for those working alone.

1. **Start by identifying a specific traumatic incident from your past.** Choose something that is at least three years old to minimize any complications from the dynamics of a current event. An example might be "the time my father punched me when I was twelve." In contrast, "my father abused me" would be too broad because, chances are, the abuse took place over many incidents. Throughout this exercise, remind yourself to stay on your original issue because it's easy to shift to other issues as you tap.

2. **Now *guess* at what your emotional intensity would be** (on the 0-to-10 scale) *if* you were to vividly imagine the incident. **Do not** actually imagine it (although

many close their eyes and do this anyway). This *guess* is a surprisingly useful estimate…and it serves to minimize emotional pain. Write your *guess* down. This guess represents your memory's emotional intensity.

3. **Next, develop a phrase to use for the EFT process,** such as "this father-punch emotion," and then proceed with a round of tapping.

4. **After this round of tapping, take another *guess*** as to what your emotional intensity about the subject is now and write it down.

5. **If your emotional intensity is still strong,** perform more rounds of EFT using the same phrase. In my experience, a total of three or four rounds will bring just about everyone down to *guesses* of 0 to 3.

6. **Perform another round of tapping** once you come down to acceptably low *guesses*. After this round, try to vividly imagine and actually relive the incident. Notice that this is the first time you are being asked to do this. All previous times have been relatively painless *guesses*. In my experience, just about everyone goes straight to zero and the rest are at very low numbers.

I urge everyone who works with trauma to try this. Try it on groups. Try it on individuals. Try it on war veterans, rape victims, and torture victims. Try it wherever trauma is involved, especially with those who are afraid of the intensity they usually feel when discussing or "getting into" their incident.

The energy based therapies have been very impressive in their ability to handle negative emotions. That is indelibly clear to practitioners using these procedures. I think the above technique, properly mastered, adds a useful component to the "art of delivery."

5

Choices, Solutions, and Tapping Tips

Dr. Patricia Carrington's "Choices" Method

Patricia Carrington, Ph.D., Associate Clinical Professor at the UMDNJ-Robert Wood Johnson Medical School in New Jersey, was one of the first clinical psychologists to incorporate EFT into her professional practice. She not only became a leading practitioner of Emotional Freedom Techniques, but she made an important contribution to its Setup Phrase. Basic or mechanical EFT focuses entirely on problems. It starts with statements like, "Even though I have this pain in my back.." or, "Even though my shoulder is in agony..." and ends with the phrase, "I deeply and completely accept myself." The treatment then proceeds with the repetition of a "problem" Reminder Phrase such as the phrase, "This pain." There's no doubt that by using this type of Setup Phrase, you can tap a problem out. But Dr. Carrington took a different approach and showed that you can also tap a *solution* in. She did this by adding "I choose" to the last portion of the Setup Phrase, making it possible for the person to define or describe a specific desired outcome by inserting an affirmation or positive statement after the words "I choose."

As she explains:

> When I was using EFT with my own clients in psychotherapy, I soon discovered that I could get even better results if I allowed them to insert their own positive affirmations into the EFT statement. This way the Setup Phrase became perfectly suited to the problems they were addressing.
>
> For example, if a person's hand was throbbing, I would suggest an EFT statement such as, "Even though my hand is throbbing, I choose to have my hand be comfortable and pain free." This immediately makes perfect sense to the injured person; it expresses precisely what they want to bring about—the cessation of pain and the healing of their hand.
>
> It was through experimenting with my own clients that the EFT Choices Method was born. In it, the person applying the method identifies the outcome that they would truly like to have for the problem at hand, and then puts this desired outcome into a phrase which they use at the end of the Setup phrase. Instead of "I deeply and completely accept myself," this phrase commences with the words "I choose."
>
> It's important to note that "I choose" is not used in the format of a traditional affirmation. The latter is a statement that is intentionally contrary to

fact, as, for example when a person living in a dingy basement apartment says, "I live in a beautiful sunny home." This statement is intentionally contrary to fact. According to the rules of traditional affirmations it will result in subconscious programming that attracts the "beautiful sunny" home of the person's dreams. All too often, however, traditional affirmations result in doubt and skepticism on the part of those who repeat them, particularly if the affirmation is in too sharp a contrast to their current state of affairs.

When people tell themselves that they live in a beautiful sunny home when in fact that is obviously not true, the traditional affirmation is apt to create what EFT refers to as a "Tail-ender." A little doubting self-statement in the back of our minds says, "Oh yeah? I know that's absurd!" or "I'll *never* have that!" or "I feel like a fool for saying this."

Such self-doubts are stilled, however, when you place the words "I choose" at the beginning of your affirmation statement. For example, if the person described above were to say, "Even though I live in a dingy basement apartment, I choose to live in a lovely sunny home," the statement would be immediately believable because anyone has the right to make a "choice" and this doesn't contradict the situation they are in.

This method of injecting "Choices" into EFT soon developed into a definite protocol which I found to be extremely effective, not only for my own clients and workshop participants, but for many others as well.

I then formalized the Choices Method and began training other people to use it. It was almost immediately greeted with enthusiasm in the EFT community, and today many thousands of people are using EFT Choices statements. In particular, psychotherapists, counselors, and personal performance coaches are using the Choices Method because it so precisely targets their clients' problems.

* * *

Dr. Carrington's six rules for phrasing Choices statements are sensible and effective:

1. Be specific.

2. Create *pulling* Choices.

3. Go for the best possible outcome.

4. State your Choices in the positive.

5. Make Choices that apply to you.

6. Make Choices that are easy to pronounce.

"Pulling Choices" use words that draw you in and make you feel involved. They are the opposite of dull and boring statements. Dr. Carrington begins with the example, "I choose to express myself in a way that gets my points across to Susan," which is a perfectly accurate statement as far as it goes. But, she says, an even more appealing version might be, "I choose to find a *creative* way to get my points across to Susan." As she explains, the word *creative* gives the statement some excitement and suspense. You wonder what would be a *creative* way to get your points across. As she says, "Curiosity is a powerful motivator." *Surprise* is another word that can draw us in, so another effective statement could be, "I choose to *surprise myself* by finding easy and enjoyable ways to get my points across to Susan." *Easy* and *enjoyable* are pulling words, too, and they help make this a compelling statement.

Here's an example of a Setup Phrase that falls short of the six recommendations:

Even though my back hurts, I choose to have it not hurt.

Following Dr. Carrington's suggestions, we can add specific details about the pain, insert some interesting or compelling ideas, describe what we'd rather have, replace negative words (no, not, can't, won't, etc.) with positive words, and create a personally rewarding Choices Phrase. For example:

Even though I have this sharp, red, throbbing, angry, hard, pyramid-shaped pain stabbing the small of my back just to the left of my spine, I choose to be delighted by how easy it is to enjoy a relaxed, pain-free game of golf tomorrow, with full range of motion, perfect coordination, and my best score yet.

Even though my back has me crying in pain, and I can't believe that this tapping business is going to make any difference at all, I choose to have this whole situation work to my advantage. I choose to have fun doing these EFT exercises in the most ingenious way, with the enthusiastic cooperation of my brilliant subconscious mind, so that the whole process is easy, comfortable, and effortless, and my back feels completely well.

While tapping on the EFT acupoints, try alternating between "problem" and "solution" Reminder Phrases.

For example, in the first round of tapping, use "problem" reminders:

Top of Head:	*stabbing pain*
Inside Eyebrow:	*so frustrating*
Side of Eye:	*terrible pain*
Under Eye:	*can't move*

and so on, through all the tapping points

Or use the same complete "problem" sentence on all of the acupoints, such as:

Top of Head:	*I'm upset because my back is in agony.*
Inside Eyebrow:	*I'm upset because my back is in agony.*
Side of Eye:	*I'm upset because my back is in agony.*

and so on, through all the tapping points.

Then, in the second round of tapping, use only positive "solution" phrases, such as:

Top of Head:	*better already*
Inside Eyebrow:	*pain-free*
Side of Eye:	*complete range of motion*
Under Eye:	*everything's easy*

and so on, through all the tapping points

Or use the same complete "solution" sentence on all of the acupoints, such as:

Top of Head:	*I choose to feel completely well in every way.*

Inside Eyebrow: *I choose to feel completely well in every way.*

Side of Eye: *I choose to feel completely well in every way.*

and so on, through all the tapping points.

In the third and final round of tapping, alternate between "problem" and "solution" phrases, such as:

Top of Head: *stabbing pain*

Inside Eyebrow: *I feel wonderful*

Side of Eye: *sharp spasms*

Under Eye: *full range of motion*

Under Nose: *so frustrating*

and so on, through all the tapping points, always ending on a "solution" phrase.

Or alternate between the two complete sentences used above:

Top of Head: *I'm upset because my back is in agony.*

Inside Eyebrow: *I choose to feel completely well in every way.*

Side of Eye: *I'm upset because my back is in agony.*

Under Eye: *I choose to feel completely well in every way.*

and so on, through all the tapping points.

To be sure your final phrase is positive (you should always end on a positive note), finish by tapping on the Inside Eyebrow point while saying a positive Reminder Phrase.

Some practitioners start with problem Reminder Phrases in the first round of tapping, alternate between problem and solution Reminder Phrases in the second, and devote the third round entirely to solution statements.

Some begin with the basic EFT Setup Phrase ("Even though _____, I fully and completely accept myself," or something similar) for their first two Setup Phrases and switch to Choices phrasing for the third Setup Phrase.

Some use only one Setup Phrase and incorporate everything in it before they start tapping the acupoints. Like EFT itself, the Choices Method is flexible, and there is no single "right" way to use it.

The Choices Method is brilliant because it helps people figure out not only what they don't want but what they do want, it installs affirmations and positive statements, and it helps speed results. Patricia Carrington is truly an EFT pioneer, and I applaud her discoveries.

Experience is the best teacher, and as you experiment with EFT, you will develop your own approach. In the mean time, tap while you read reports about EFT sessions that work. This simple practice will help you incorporate many different approaches into your EFT repertoire.

When EFT Doesn't Work

EFT can work in the most extreme conditions, when many factors could be expected to interfere with its success, so there are no hard and fast rules about when and where it will work and where it won't. But from time to time conditions do interfere. The following are common problems that are easily corrected. If you find that EFT isn't working—you or the person you're working with experience no change and the situation seems stuck—try these remedies.

1. **There may be a problem with energy in the room,** or you may be exposed to an energy toxin. Try going outside or into another room. There are many possible sources of electromagnetic interference, including fluorescent lighting. An easy way to help clear your mind and body is to go outdoors and stand for several minutes with your bare feet on bare ground, grass, sand, concrete, or rocks. The earth supplies a constant supply of free electrons, which are anti-inflammatory and help balance energy. Wearing shoes, being indoors, and riding in cars insulates us from those free electrons.

    Our modern lifestyles also deprive us of full-spectrum natural light, which our endocrine systems need in order to function well. To remedy that problem, spend as much time as possible outdoors, on a screened porch, or near an open window or doorway—without wearing sunglasses, reading glasses, or contact lenses, all of which prevent the transmission of full-spectrum light. A shady location is fine so long as your eyes have access to natural light.

    In addition, being outdoors (assuming the air quality is reasonable) provides fresh air and oxygen. Take several deep breaths, really filling your lungs. Then try your Setup Phrase and tapping sequence again.

2. **Maybe it's something you ate.** A few years ago I worked with a woman who had suffered major bouts of depression since age nine. When I first met her, Louella was suicidal. Tears came easily and "hopeless" seemed to be her favorite word. EFT tapping

helped, but whenever her depression lifted a little, it came right back—and this continued after we found and treated several core issues, relieving her back pain and asthma along the way.

During our sixth partially successful session, she felt better until she ate an apple. Within minutes she was on the brink of a panic attack, her depression shot back to a 10, she acted as though she had taken a drug, and she fell asleep for several hours.

We invented a "detective diet" to establish what other foods might be causing her problem. She agreed to eat only organic foods (the apple that put her to sleep was not organically grown), eat one food at a time, and wait one hour between foods.

From the moment Louella started this detective diet, her depression began to lift, and within 24 hours it completely disappeared. She began sleeping normally, went on long hikes with friends, enjoyed dancing again, and vacationed in Spain. She learned to avoid wheat, which was the only organic food that triggered an adverse reaction. As long as she stayed away from wheat and commercially grown fruits and vegetables, she felt terrific.

Louella's food sensitivities are not unusual. Many holistic physicians routinely recommend that their patients stop eating common allergens, like wheat and dairy products, and in many cases their health improves right away.

Many EFTers notice that when they eat certain foods, they soon feel tired, their memory declines, simple projects seem suddenly complicated, and even the simplest EFT tapping requires exhausting effort. In fact, many forget all about EFT. Responses to food are individual, but many experience this kind of fatigue soon after they eat sweets and other carbohydrates.

3. **Try varying the Setup Phrase.** Try switching from the Karate Chop point to the Sore Spot for your set-up phrase, or vice versa.

   Also, your set-up phrase may be too general, too global. Make it more specific. Focus on a single incident or a single upsetting detail in an incident. By alternating between the Sore Spot and Karate Chop point and by focusing on the details of upsetting past events, you'll make rapid progress.

4. **You may not know what to tap for.** This is not unusual, especially for beginners. It's hard to know what issue to choose, which detail to select, or how to address an issue once you find it. Your subconscious mind can be your ally here. Try using a Setup Phrase that invites the subconscious mind to communicate, such as:

   Even though I don't know how to use EFT for this problem, I know that my imagination will come up with an appropriate phrase.

Even though I don't know how to define this problem, the right words will come to me without effort.

Even though I can't think right now, I know that deep within me my clever, intelligent mind understands exactly what I hope to accomplish, and it is organizing my thoughts in the best possible way for a good outcome.

5. **You may need to do more repetitions.** I often say that the secrets to success with EFT are focus and perseverance. As long as you experience at least some improvement, you are moving in the right direction. EFT practitioners and students often report that when they felt stuck, going nowhere, but continued to tap and tap and tap—suddenly everything shifted.

6. **You may be avoiding unhappy memories.** Some people feel uncomfortable saying negative Setup Phrases. They're afraid that thinking about a problem will make it worse. This fear is actually a wonderful tapping subject. By focusing on their fear of tapping, many EFT novices have jumped straight to core issues with excellent results. Example: *I don't want to tap on my weight problem.*

There's your opportunity! Start tapping on:

Even though I don't want to tap on my weight problem, it makes me uncomfortable, I'd rather not even think about it, I don't want to do this, I don't want to think about ＿＿＿＿＿＿, and I definitely don't want to remember ＿＿＿＿＿.

Let your mind fill in the blanks. Unhappy memories are what make EFT work. Welcome those unhappy memories and start tapping.

EFT is not designed to be a painful procedure. Just tap and think about an unhappy event from a distance, then move a little closer. If it begins to feel painful, back up and tap until the feeling subsides. Then continue. Thanks to EFT tapping, you won't have to relive the experience. You can observe it from a distance without being emotionally involved. This step-by-step procedure, which we call the Tearless Trauma Technique, has freed EFTers of all ages from the shackles of painful memories while neutralizing core issues that created their pain and discomfort.

7. **Try tapping more often.** Try to tap at least five times a day—and more often when you think of it. Set a tapping goal, such as tapping every hour on the hour or at a certain time of day. Tap while you read this book. Find a tapping buddy, someone who can tap with you in person or on the phone, and tap with that person at every opportunity. Recruit friends or family members to form a tapping group. Tap while you watch TV. Tap while you walk the dog. Tap before every meal, whenever you use the bathroom, and whenever you take a bath or shower. Serious EFTers are ingenious about creating time to tap throughout the day.

8. **Look for new perspectives.** Always try to find a new way of looking at an old, stuck issue. This book introduces many different ways of describing pain. Approach your problem from new directions. Involve your imagination. Think of the problem as a play or movie and put your favorite actors in the cast. Think of it as a computer game and visualize its special effects. Go back to the Personal Peace Procedure and work through a dozen different issues.

9. **Watch yourself in a mirror as you tap.** Mirror tapping is an excellent way to discover phrases and statements that make you feel uncomfortable. For example, some are able to say "I fully and completely accept and love myself" if they're looking at a wall but not if they're looking at themselves in a mirror. Once EFT neutralizes negative emotions and you install positive emotions and affirmations in their place, mirror tapping can strengthen those positive results, making them a more powerful part of you.

10. **Shout it out!** If the set-up phrase isn't getting through, you may not be saying it loudly enough. In many of my seminars, I've had people *shout* their set-up phrases. Some people do this in their cars with the radio volume turned up. Others do it in the shower. To involve your entire being in this exercise, use emphatic gestures or jump up and down.

11. **Get some vigorous exercise.** There's a definite connection between the lymph system and the body's energy system. When you're sedentary, lymph doesn't circulate, so the body's waste removal slows down,

and that interferes with not only EFT but your overall health and thought processes. Some exciting EFT results have been achieved immediately after a vigorous physical workout. Try jogging, going for a hike, swimming as fast as you can, bouncing on a rebounder (miniature trampoline), or riding a bike immediately before your next tapping session.

12. **Clear your energy.** Donna Eden, author of the best seller *Energy Medicine* and co-author (with David Feinstein and me) of *The Promise of Energy Psychology,* has taught thousands how to clear their energy and keep it balanced with tapping and other exercises. See any of Donna's books or videos for instructions.

Try all of these techniques and keep track of your results so you'll know which strategies work best for you.

EFT instructor Barbara Smith wrote the following for our email newsletter. She makes several helpful observations.

What to Do When EFT Doesn't Work

by Barbara Smith

Have you ever thought, "I tried that EFT and it didn't work," or, "How is it that I am tapping all this time and getting so nowhere?" If you have temporarily faltered in your EFT journey, these tips are for you.

1. The One-minute Wonder.

Sometimes, when we first learn EFT, we are fortunate enough to experience or watch one of those amazing demonstrations that result in profound, and seemingly instant, change. We refer to these as a One-Minute Wonders. They are so exciting and satisfying. They seem so easy and so effective. No wonder people talk about EFT as the best thing since sliced bread. This kind of transforming success can build our expectation that every session will be like that. When we try it out at home on our own and the problem does not instantly resolve, we feel disappointed and discouraged. We may wonder if there is something the matter with us. Sometimes we lose heart and give up.

The one-minute wonders that you see in demonstrations do happen, but not all the time. Trainers who work with groups are usually very experienced and able to employ a range of sophisticated EFT techniques. Good trainers make intuitive judgments about which issue to address, the language to use, and the best technique for the situation. You as a Newbie are still learning the basics. Keep tapping until the process becomes second nature.

2. When EFT Hasn't Worked *Yet.*

It would be easy to head this paragraph "EFT doesn't work for me." This is what disappointed clients say. But when I reframe it as "EFT hasn't worked YET," I shift our focus away from failure and we can hold the "yet" as a positive intention.

The metaphor that guides me here and the one I use most frequently is the image of water dripping on a stone. It might take a while to see the effect, but every time EFT "doesn't work," we learn another lesson about ourselves and about what works and what doesn't work for each situation.

3. Do EFT for EFT.

When someone tells me that he or she forgot to use EFT at home, or decided not to use it, we might discuss the reasons, and the client may promise to "try harder." At that point, I suggest that tapping now would be useful, and that we will do EFT for EFT.

Even though this tapping stuff isn't working, I fully and completely accept myself...

Even though I forget to do EFT when it would be really useful....

Even though I have messed it up...

Even though I give up on EFT before I'm fully over the problem...

When we have lowered our discomfort, frustration, or anxiety about the EFT not working, we will be free to address the next layer of presenting issues. We may even find some specific events involving our own beliefs about success, and we would tap for those. This meta-level of tapping can be very useful.

4. The "Felt" Experience.

One of the ways we know that EFT is really working for us is through "felt" experience. Most adults do not notice the changes in skin temperature, the constant shifts of muscle tension, and the tightness or lack of muscle tone at any moment. When the EFT seems not to be working, you have probably forgotten to notice what is happening in your body.

It is very useful to stop and notice exactly what has changed. Has the tension gone out of your chest, are your shoulders tense or relaxed, or has the mental picture changed? Does your body feel lighter, your breath easier? Has the thought changed? Teach yourself to notice these changes using all of your senses. Later, you can refer back to the specific experience to find what you might be overlooking or to recapture the feeling of success that you previously discovered.

5. EFT Will Never Work for Me.

There are some situations where beginners can give up or feel hopeless. There are many reasons that may stop you from reaching instant success. One reason is psychological reversal. When we first learn EFT, we begin to work on ourselves using the basic skills. We don't have enough experience and confidence to treat some deeper issues. This is the time to work one-to-one, in person, by phone, or in a group, with an experienced practitioner who is familiar with the more sophisticated applications of EFT and who will help you recognize and address core experiences and hidden beliefs that may block you from change.

6. What Words Were You Using?

When people tell me that the EFT didn't work, I ask for specific information about the issue, its aspects, and the phrases the client was saying. This is the way to get specific about what happened or where the protocol might be improved. Write down the issue, the Reminder Phrase you are using, and the intensity level of your distress in relation to this issue. This is especially important if you are working on your own. Note every change in aspect, and/or intensity after each round. In this way, you will be able to look back and remind yourself of your progress and previous successes. If you are helping someone else with EFT, this record will ensure you can quickly identify any issues that may have been overlooked.

7. Too Much Too Fast?

Because EFT is not working at home does not mean that EFT will not work. It just means it has not worked—yet. Sometime the reason is that we have tried to address one of our truly big issues, one whose distress level is overwhelming. Try some practice sessions on less intense issues, or choose a less arousing aspect of your problem before going back to the *big one.*

8. The EFT Skeptics' Society.

Most of us have had years of experience of using the thinking-talking-trying harder process of therapeutic change, and in the beginning we may find ourselves drifting back to a talk model, because we find it very difficult to believe that something as strange as EFT will really work.

Those of us who are health professionals know that many of our colleagues are still skeptical about EFT. I remember that it took me some time before I routinely used EFT on myself. I chose a few colleagues with whom to share what I was learning, and gradually I became more confident about presenting EFT to others.

Now I use it on everything and cannot imagine how I ever lived without EFT.

Find a friend, colleague or professional who knows and uses EFT. If you don't know any EFT person near you, arrange some telephone coaching, subscribe to an EFT newsletter, and read accounts from others about their success with EFT. Keep up to date with innovations through internet newsletters. Support may be the very thing that makes the difference.

Once you have achieved a high rate of success with EFT in your own life, other people's skepticism really does not matter. You can change your response to others with a little tapping: *Even though I really hate the way she rolls her eyes when I mention EFT...*

9.   Testing, Testing, Testing.

Are you testing at home? What are you testing? In my practice this is the thing that new clients find the most difficult to do consistently at home. Is it possible that you wandered off target?

Before you decide that EFT is not working for you, write down your distress level and the problem's aspects for every round. Some issues take several rounds before they completely clear. I suggest to my clients that if they think there is no change, they should be prepared to do up to five rounds at any one level of intensity before they move to a new aspect or topic. If you carefully record your intensity rate and are clear about the aspect you're treating, you will probably find yourself making progress.

10. Back to Basics with "The EFT Course."

The EFT Course is presented in Gary Craig's EFT Manual and introductory DVDs. The EFT manual remains the definitive source of EFT theory and practice. Experienced therapists have been integrating EFT with many other psychological and physiological forms of healing, while others have been creating variations that we sometimes call EFT"s "cousins." If EFT is not working for you, check to be sure that you are following all of the EFT basics in your sessions at home.

Then, in the words of family therapist Virginia Satir, *"Try it on everything and swallow only what fits."*

✦ ✦ ✦

6

EFT in Action
for Back Pain

There are so many ways in which EFT has relieved pain that it's impossible to describe them all, but thanks to reports from EFT practitioners and instructors, I have many examples to share. Tap your EFT points while you read these descriptions, and when you come across a story that resonates with you, try inserting your own situation and see what happens.

Here, from EFT instructor Maggie Adkins, are three approaches that can help you explore your pain.

Three Methods for Working with Pain
by Maggie Adkins

There are numerous ways to work with pain using EFT. Sometimes pain just shifts while you are working on another issue. That issue could be anything—past trauma; anger; grief; sadness, or a myriad of other issues. At other times, you may want to do

EFT while focused specifically on pain. Here are three ways to work with pain in the body.

1. **Focus on the actual pain.**

    Even though I have this lightning bolt pain in my side...

    Even though I have this throbbing headache in the front of my head...

    Even though I have this dull ache in my left knee...

2. **Focus on how you feel about the pain.**

    Even though I'm afraid if this pain keeps up, I won't be able to dance anymore...

    Even though I'm terrified I'll lose my job if this pain gets worse...

    Even though if I were the person I think I am, I would have gotten rid of this pain long ago...

    Even though I have these emotions about having this pain...

3. **Find an emotion or quality in the pain or part of the body in pain.**

    Even though I have this resentment in my shoulder....

    Even though I have this anger in my lower back —nobody ever supported me and I'm tired of doing it all myself...

    Even though I have this shame/grief/sadness (whatever it is) in my back...

These are just a few ideas. Use your genius and your intuition.

❀ ❀ ❀

Now we'll take a look at some of those famous EFT One-Minute Wonders. The first is from Graham Batchelor, who runs a sports injury clinic in the UK and who was astonished at how well EFT helped his client's severe pain from a back injury.

Pain from Severe Lower Back Injury Resolved

by Graham Batchelor

Your free introduction manual to EFT whetted my appetite and I so ordered your DVD package. It arrived very quickly into the UK, and I became so enthralled that I spent almost all my time over the next 14 days engrossed in the material. I must confess I did neglect my sports injury clinic but something told me that EFT was the way forward and the more knowledge I could gain, the better my results with treatments would be.

This was proven to be correct when an appointment was made by a 45-year-old gentleman who told me that following a serious injury to his lower back at work, he was hospitalized for six months and confined to a wheelchair for a further two years. Physiotherapists had worked with him over this period and eventually got him walking with the aid of two crutches, but he was only able to cover about 30 meters (100 feet) at a time. Although he was on powerful analgesics, he still suffered a large amount of pain, and he was told that little more could be done for him. He made an appointment for the next day.

When he arrived, I could tell from his efforts to walk that his lower back and legs were pain-ridden. His posture was very lopsided, and he was completely exhausted from the efforts to get to me. He found it very difficult to get onto the treatment couch but insisted on doing so.

Although I had only just gained a small under-standing of EFT, I began talking through the prob-lems he had faced since the injury. It became obvious that he felt exceptionally guilty about his inability to help his wife when cancer struck and she underwent a major operation. He was also concerned that his earn-ing power had dropped to zero. He indicated his qual-ity of life was only a 2 on the "positive" 0-to-10 scale.

I gained his permission to try EFT with him and began with the Karate Chop point. We went through a basic setup procedure using:

> *Even though I have this serious injury…*
>
> *Even though I could not help my wife in her time of urgent need…*
>
> *Even though I can no longer support my family…*

When we reached the collarbone point, he began sobbing, his breathing became labored, and his lower body began twitching. We stopped and I explained that I thought he was going through a very strong emotional release. He gradually regained composure and we carried on.

At the end of the second round he requested that we continue, indicating he felt much better emotionally and his pain was reducing. After the third round I prepared to help him off the couch. Amazingly, he stood by himself and, using only one stick, began walking around the treatment room.

I advised him not to be too adventurous and to take things a little easy. With tears of happiness in his eyes, he could not thank me enough. I explained that EFT and he himself were the healers and I was only a channel. Talking through his treatment, he now said he felt his quality of life had gone to a wonderful 9 out of 10 and he could not wait to get home to his wife. I talked to him and his wife three days later and neither could believe his recovery.

After running a sports injury clinic using shiatsu, Reiki, and other healing techniques for almost 20 years, I cannot believe how EFT helped this patient. I intend to use it at every opportunity. I look forward to getting much more experience and understanding, but for this first attempt, I truly am amazed.

✾ ✾ ✾

Graham was concerned about his client's welfare when he warned him not to do too much now that he felt better, but I agree with Dr. Sarno that as soon as we let go of the emotional factors that keep us in pain, we can safely resume of our normal activities. EFT is always available as a first-aid treatment if we need it.

Doing EFT over the phone can be highly effective, as is clearly illustrated in this report by seasoned EFTer Aileen Nobles.

Eight Months of Chronic Back Pain Disappears
by Aileen Nobles

When I spoke to Joanie on the phone she was terrified and desperate. She was in so much pain, and yet so afraid of having a session that she had previously canceled me twice. The third time she kept her phone appointment. She suffered from chronic pain down the right side of her neck and shoulder, down her back and into her arm and hand. This pain had been going on for eight months and she told me she had only had a couple of hours sleep a night for many months. She had not been able to work, was depressed and she was at her wits' end. Her pain level was consistently at a 9 or 10 on a scale of 0-to-10.

When I asked her what happened in her life around eight months ago she couldn't remember anything of importance. I explained that our bodies have almost unlimited restorative healing capabilities if there is a free flow of energy in the meridians. Whenever our physical body is feeling less than perfect, it is asking us to look at our emotional body. Something had probably happened around the time this pain started.

Intuitively I knew that working on the pain alone was not going to produce the change I wanted. The fact that she had canceled me twice and was so afraid led me to believe some kind of emotional trauma was being suppressed. Again I asked her if anything out of the ordinary had happened eight months ago when this pain started. She couldn't think of anything.

I mentioned that even though she couldn't think of anything right now her subconscious and super conscious were both holding the necessary information. I suggested we start tapping and we would see if anything came up.

Even though I can't remember what happened eight months ago...

Even though part of me may be afraid to remember if anything happened that was very upsetting, I'm still quite wonderful anyway.

We moved to the gamut point and tapped on:

My subconscious knows if anything happened, and my super conscious is always protecting me.

I would like to believe that I am in safe hands, and it's safe for me to bring any situation connected with my pain into my conscious mind.

Bingo! Joanie blurted out that eight months ago her mother died! Yes, that was a painful experience! Joanie's mother had always been a strong support system, helping Joanie to believe in herself. She depended on her mother so much that she had always been afraid that without her mother she wouldn't want to live. Joanie was married to a very sweet and gentle man, and when her mother crossed over she didn't want him to know that she felt like dying. She didn't want him to feel that her mother meant more to her than his love for her.

She had so much internal pain connected with the loss of her support system—her mother—and guilt over not wanting to hurt her husband that she stuffed it all inside. She chose not to deal with it to the point of blocking it out...but her physical body had other ideas. We tapped on:

My husband loves me so much he does not want me to be in pain and its okay to talk to him about how much I miss my mother.

I'm safe and loved and he will understand how I feel.

Now that I am safe enough to acknowledge my inner pain, it no longer needs to manifest as outer pain.

Thank you wonderful physical body for bringing my attention to emotions that needed to be addressed.

We did a few rounds on releasing the sadness.

I have a lot if pain inside as I miss my mother so much.

Joanie then held the points under her eyes without tapping. *My pain on the inside is manifesting on the outside, I'd like to let it go.* She took three deep breaths. *My pain on the inside no longer needs to manifest on the outside as I allow myself to release it.* She took three more deep breaths, and we began to reframe the loss. Joanie acknowledged that her mother would not want her to be sad and in pain, and being sad wasn't accomplishing anything useful. Her mother would want her to become strong and enjoy her wonderful husband. We continued tapping:

The last thing my mother would want is for me to be in pain.

My mother always wanted me to be happy with my husband.

Joanie's level of pain was now down to 2 out of 10 and was in her neck. We continued tapping:

Even though I have this two pain in my neck I really am terrific anyway.

Even if this pain in my neck is me, I'm still quite wonderful anyway.

I don't need to be a pain in the neck to myself or anyone else, I'm ready to heal and be happy and productive.

She laughed out loud and said the pain was all gone, and she was looking forward to speaking openly with her husband. Joanie no longer had any guilt connected with not loving her husband enough, as she accepted how we love different people differently. Her love for her husband was very special in its own unique way.

We talked about her going back to work and feeling as if she had a purpose, she was so amazed and excited that she was pain free and felt so differently than she had at the beginning of the phone call. She did start working again with her husband and is still pain free.

Again and again I see pain and illness lift and disappear even when painkillers are not having any effect. What an incredible tool we have in our own hands.

❊ ❊ ❊

It isn't every day that attorneys relieve their clients of back pain. Notice how attorney Ted Robinson aims EFT at emotional issues to clear up his client's pain. Notice also how the client tries to "explain away" the result. This often happens with astonished newcomers to EFT. They have a hard time believing that fingertip tapping could have such immediate and profound effects.

Attorney Relieves Client's Back Pain

by Ted Robinson

I was with a young woman who was charged with two felonies for forging a prescription for oxycodone, which she said she had to do because of severe back pain after an auto accident. She claimed her insurance ran out and the doctor wouldn't give her any more prescriptions, so she arranged to have some blanks given to her and she forged them to get her pain relievers. She said she had a ruptured disc between L-4/L-5. Of course, as soon as we left the court, I suggested we give EFT a try.

Her 0-to-10 intensity was a 6 or 7. Then after a simple set-up of "this pain in my back that's a 7," I started the sequence with "This pain in my back" and repeated it as we went through the points. I was shortly drawn to add other wording like,

Even though I'm carrying my whole family around on my back…

Even though it's not fair…

Even though I have the entire responsibility for our entire family on my shoulders and back…

Within about 90 seconds I noticed her moving her back to check to see if it still hurt. Her expression was somewhat quizzical and she looked at me and said, "It feels better … much better. But you made me think about all that tapping instead of my back, right?"

I said no, it was just the energy being balanced and the underlying issues being recognized. She was much happier and relieved knowing she had a new way to deal with her pain. She also realized that if she had such a method ahead of time, she never would have been arrested or be facing jail time.

❀ ❀ ❀

Here is another EFT phone session that alleviated back pain.

Three-week Back Pain Relieved in Phone Session

by CJ Puotinen

While confirming registrations for an upcoming workshop, I left a phone message for Holly Anne Shelowitz, a nutrition counselor in Kingston, NY. When Holly called back, she explained that she hadn't replied to my emails because she hadn't been able to access her computer for three weeks. She had injured her back and had been in bed that whole time. Friends were staying with her in shifts 24 hours a day because she needed help doing everything. Every movement was excruciatingly painful.

"I don't know anything about EFT," she said, "but I was wondering if there is some way I can get started now, before the workshop, in case it would help with the pain."

I asked her to describe the pain, beginning with its size, shape, and location. She said it had at first covered her entire back, but it was now in the small of her back. In response to my questions (is it bigger than a breadbox, is it square or round, what is its three-dimensional shape, is it soft or hard, is it smooth or rough, what color is it, does it make a sound, does it move or pulse) she described it as the size and shape of a slightly squashed grapefruit, red-orange in color, with a hard spiky, thorny surface, not making any noise, and not moving or pulsing.

We slowly went through the EFT tapping points. She used a phone headset, which freed her hands for tapping, and soon she was tapping along at a good clip, saying,

Even though there's a pain in the small of my back that's the size and shape of a slightly squashed hard red-orange grapefruit, and it's covered with thorns and spikes, and it's just stuck there and it won't move except to cause a lot of pain whenever I move, and it has turned me into an invalid, in fact I'm a total mess, I fully and completely accept myself.

Even though this pain is overwhelming and it's kept me flat on my back for three weeks and my back is a mess and my life is a mess, I fully and completely accept myself, I love and forgive myself, I forgive this pain, I forgive my back, and I choose to be pleasantly surprised at how easy it is to relax and let go of this pain and feel better.

Even though this tapping business is very strange, I'm desperate enough to try anything, and who knows, maybe it will unblock some blocked energy and let my meridians flow the way they're supposed to, and maybe I'll feel a little better in a few minutes.

These statements were interspersed with the EFT point tapping, starting at the top of her head, the third eye at the center of her forehead, inside eyebrow, outside eye, under the eye, under the nose, under the lip, collar bone, under the arm, and several taps across the upper abdomen. My husband's Tibetan acupuncturist suggested that rather than focus on a specific liver point, we tap all over the upper abdomen, from waist to part way up the rib cage and from far right to far left, because several meridians run through that area, and the more places we tap, the more likely we are to hit meridians that will help.

At each tapping point, I had Holly say a different Reminder Phrase: *pain, hurts, red-orange, hard, spiky, thorns, rough, hard, difficult, squashed grapefruit, etc.*

After a few quick rounds of head-to-torso tapping, Holly sounded more relaxed. I assumed that her pain was diminishing, but I wanted to give her a good foundation for future reference, so instead of asking how she felt, I taught her the hand points, explaining that she might not need them but it's good to know how to use them just in case. We completed the finger tapping by tapping the fingertips of the right hand against the nails of the left hand, and vice versa.

After a few rounds that incorporated the hand points, we did the 9 Gamut treatment. I called it the "brain-balancer" and explained that it brings the left and right brains into balance. Holly was happy to learn this simple procedure.

Then I asked Holly how she felt about the pain. Soon she was saying, while tapping on her karate chop point,

Even though I'm furious with this pain, totally angry and upset, here I am stuck in bed, not able to work, not able to go anywhere, not able to do anything by myself, dependent on everyone, it's so frustrating, my body betrayed me, I have no control over my body or anything, it's so upsetting!

Even though I hate all this, I fully and completely accept myself, I love and forgive myself, I forgive myself for hurting my back, I forgive my back for being hurt, I forgive anyone and anything that had anything to do with my being in this condition, and I choose to amaze myself at how easy it is to let go of this hard, thorny, excruciating red-orange spiky pain, to let it go, to release it and everything that has contributed to it in any way, and I choose to be completely well, I choose to let my body heal itself from the inside, I choose to relax and be happy, and that's the truth!

Tap tap tap tap tap with appropriate Reminder Phrases: *angry, frustrated, body betrayed me, upset, etc.,* followed in the next round by positive Reminder Phrases: *let go, release, forgive, love, good back, strong back, happy back.*

Just to be sure we were clearing everything that might be a factor, I started Holly on a new Setup Phrase, saying,

Here I am stuck in bed, I've been here for three weeks, life is passing me by while I stare at the ceiling, I may be here forever, and I find, as I lie here thinking about everything, that this reminds me of _____.

Holly stopped, then realized that I was waiting for her to fill in the blank. "This reminds me of when I had an infected tooth," she said, "and I was lying in the dentist's chair with all that cotton and stuff in my mouth, totally helpless, not in control of anything, not able to move because of a condition I could do nothing to fix. It was the most awful feeling. I was afraid and upset and helpless, and I think feeling helpless is what bothered me the most."

So we tapped on:

Even though I feel helpless, just as helpless as when I was stuck in the dentist's chair, and even though I have to rely on friends for help to do everything because I'm helpless, and even though I can't do anything for myself, can't work, can't walk, can't sit up, can't do anything by myself or for myself, I'm as helpless as a baby, I'm paralyzed, I'm stuck, I'm helpless, nevertheless I fully and completely accept myself, I love myself, I love my back, I forgive myself and my back and everything and everyone for anything and everything, and I choose to be completely well, I choose to release all this and let it go, I choose to say goodbye to the pain.

I know that in some way this pain that has kept me in bed for three weeks was my body's attempt to keep me safe, so with gratitude I thank the part of me that controls this pain, I love and bless it, I acknowledge its excellent work, it has done its job very well, and now that it realizes that the useful purpose it served is now complete, it can let go now, right now, and it can know how much I appreciate its good work. It can come back when it's needed and necessary, and for now it can let the pain subside, it can release the pain, it can let go while I thank it for doing such a good job. I choose to be delighted at how easy it is to let the pain go, and the part of me that controls the pain can thoroughly enjoy how easy it is to release this pain now. I thank this pain, I bless this pain, and I release this pain now.

At the end of all this, Holly sighed a deep, deep sigh, a good sign that her energy was shifting. And now when she laughed, it wasn't a nervous pain-filled laugh, it was a relaxed laugh, a laugh with relief and a spark of hope and joy in it.

I asked Holly whether her pain was still the size and shape of a slightly squashed grapefruit.

"No!" she exclaimed. "It's a little cube, like a small box, and it isn't red-orange any more, it's a deep velvet blue, and it isn't rough and spiny any more, it has a smooth velvet surface. It's almost gone!"

Now we tapped on:

Even though I have this small velvet blue box of pain in the small of my back, I fully and completely love and accept myself. Even though there is still a little box of blue velvet pain in the small of my back, the pain is disappearing, it is going away, my body is healing itself from the inside out, I feel better already, I feel so much better, I really feel completely well.

At the end of two or three rounds of tapping, Holly couldn't find the pain at all. It had disappeared.

"Okay," I said, "let's see if we can find it again. Do you feel like sitting up?"

Holly realized that she probably could, and she did. I asked her to bend to the left, right, forward, and back to see if she could find the pain, and she couldn't. It was gone.

"Feel like standing up?" I asked.

"Oh, gosh," said Holly. "Do you think I should? I mean, do you think I can?"

"Well," I said, "your friend is there to help."

Her friend had in fact been rolling his eyes as he watched Holly tap and talk, but now he had something useful to do, so he stood beside her as she took a tentative move toward standing.

"I can't!" she cried and sat back. But it was not pain that interfered this time, it was fear. We tapped on:

Even though I'm afraid to stand, I feel dizzy, I'm afraid I'll fall, I think I'll faint, I'm afraid I'll injure myself all over again and I'll be right back where I started. I'm afraid this won't work. I'm afraid to try. I'm too afraid to think straight. On the other hand, I trust my strong, healthy body, which is healing itself from the inside out. I trust my brilliant mind, which is directing all my nerves and muscles to stand me up straight and keep me there. I love and trust my body and mind and nerves and bones and muscles and everything else. I choose to let go of the fear. I'm going to stand up now.

And she did! Holly was amazed. She kept laughing. "I can't believe it! I'm standing up! It was so easy!" And she couldn't find the pain, even when she leaned to the left, right, forward, and back, and even when she bent her right leg and pulled it toward her, then did the same with her left leg. She felt a little stiff from all that bed rest, but we tapped on the stiffness and she soon felt more limber.

Then she said, sounding shy and tentative, like a little girl, "It's such a beautiful day, it's so lovely outside, I wonder—do you think that maybe—could I maybe—do you think I could, well, could I go for a walk? Outside? By the lake?"

I burst out laughing. "Tap with me," I said.

Even though I've spent the last half hour lying on my back, tapping on my head, and saying all kinds of ridiculous things with someone I've never met in my life, and now I'm asking this total stranger who's 70 miles away for permission to go for a walk? Do I need my head examined?

We zipped through the tapping points, saying,

Going for a walk! I feel terrific! Going outside! Beautiful day! The end! Goodbye!

Holly and her friend took a 20-minute walk by the lake, and she felt completely fine. She immediately resumed her work and her normal activities. Nearly two years have passed since Holly's introduction to EFT, and during that entire time she has felt only an occasional minor twinge of pain, especially when she's under stress. Whenever that happens, she taps and the pain disappears.

❊ ❊ ❊

7

EFT as First Aid

Some of my favorite reports are from Newbies and experienced EFTers who use tapping as a first-aid treatment. As the following examples show, this can be an effective strategy for old injuries as well as accidents or episodes of back strain or pain that just occurred. In this next example, the client was a newcomer to EFT who used it on herself. No outside assistance was involved or needed.

Back Pain Subsides after 14 Years

by Evelia A. Sanchez

Fourteen years ago, my friend was hit by a bus and was left with terrible neck and back problems. She was in so much pain that she would go into spasms during which she could move only by hobbling and dragging one leg.

She went to many different doctors and healers but found only temporary relief for her now-crooked back and disabling pain. Her best relief came from a chiropractic treatment, but the results were only temporary and she had to go every one to three months. She did this for the last 13 years. It was terribly expensive for a woman on a small pension.

When I realized that EFT could help her, I taught it to her. I instructed her to do the work as often as she could and to let me know what happened. That was a year ago and I am proud to let everyone know that she has not needed a back adjustment in all that time.

For the first month she tapped every time she was in pain. Her back shifted quickly and the pain shifted dramatically. She could feel tingles go up and down her spine as she worked on it and that's how she knew something was changing.

She continued to go to the chiropractor just to monitor her back with X-rays, but she has not needed to have her back adjusted since starting EFT. She says that on her last visit the doctor told her that her back was almost perfectly aligned. He was so happy to report this, and he believes it was his work that helped her.

I begged her to tell him about EFT but she says he is not open to it and she does not want to offend him. Oh, well. We know the truth and he has documented it for us. Great job, EFT!

※ ※ ※

In the following case, Peggy Lawson uses EFT to relieve her dentist's substantial back pain. In the process, she "borrows benefits" and reduces her own dental pain and discomfort. Borrowing benefits is one of the many advantages we receive when we tap on behalf of others. Your own circumstances, whatever they are, improve without conscious effort on your part. How's that for a win-win situation?

How I Fixed My Dentist's Back Pain

by Peggy Lawson

I had an appointment at the dentist the other day. He had already cancelled a previous appointment because he had hurt his back.

When I arrived at his office, the dental assistant informed me that he was still in a lot of pain, but he was working because he didn't want to disappoint any more of his patients. When the dentist walked in, I could see the pain in his eyes. It occurred to me that I truly didn't want anyone who was in that much pain working in my mouth.

I asked him if he could think of any emotional reason for the pain in his back and he said, *"No, I don't think so. And it's not exactly in my back, it's more in my, ahem, lower left cheek."*

When I asked him if he was willing to allow me to show him something that might help him, he recoiled and said, *"Will it hurt?"* My eyes slid over to the huge syringe with the four-inch needle that he was preparing to stick in my jaw, and I dryly replied, *"Not as much as that's going to hurt me!"*

He was desperate and willing to try anything. So I sat up in the chair, and we did four rounds of EFT.

> *Even though my lower back hurts…*
>
> *Even though I have this pain in my left cheek…*

Finally I said:

> *Even though I have a big pain in my ass…*

Which, after two rounds, left him chuckling, but more importantly, pain-free. Free to work on me next! This next part is incredible to me.

I don't have any phobias about going to the dentist, but it's not something I look forward to, either. I hate when the needle goes into my jaw, and I really dislike the way the numbness makes my lips feel ten sizes larger and I can't even tell if I'm drooling or not. The numbness taking its time to wear off is very unpleasant also, and I sometimes bite the inside of my mouth until it does. I had none of that!

I didn't even feel the needle going into my gum, and I never felt any pain or any unpleasant numb feeling. It was if I hadn't needed an anesthetic at all. It was amazing to me. Apparently, since I had spent several minutes tapping for and with him, I borrowed the benefits of EFT from the dentist! I can't remember when that's ever happened to me before, and I tap on a lot of people!

I highly recommend tapping on your dentist next time it's necessary to go, if he or she will let you, and see if it doesn't help you!

* * *

In this next example, Dr. Larry Stewart was about to call for an ambulance when his wife pinched a nerve in her back. Thanks to EFT, the ambulance wasn't needed.

EFT Cancels an Ambulance Call

by Dr. Larry Stewart

Two weeks ago, at 8:00 on Saturday morning, I awakened to hear my wife's cries of pain. Shirley had picked up a stack of magazines and in the process had pinched a nerve in her back (she's done it before) and was lying on the ground, crying from the pain. I started to call an ambulance, but I decided to see if I could offer some immediate relief from some of the pain. She rated the pain in her back as a solid 10 and the numbness in her toes rated an 8 on the big toe and 10 on the small ones.

We tapped, but no change. We tapped again, and she felt a little relief. About 15 rounds of tapping, she was down to a 1 on the back pain, a zero on the numbness in her big toe, and a 2 or 3 on the numbness in her smaller toes. She rested and continued to tap every few hours through the weekend. We finally got her to her physician and chiropractor on Monday.

For the next few days, anytime the pain crept up, she would tap. She continued to tap for the numbness. Ten days later, she is able to walk normally again. Whenever this happened before, it meant days in bed followed by months of pain and numbness. I'm convinced that EFT helped, at least to relieve the neuro-muscular tension that accompanied the injury.

✾ ✾ ✾

From time to time we receive reports from EFTers who are injured in car crashes and other mishaps, describing how tapping reduced their pain, kept them calm, and helped them cope with whatever happened before and after the accident. When Barbara Cohn totaled her car, the first thing she did was focus on EFT.

EFT and My Car Crash

by Barbara Cohn

Day before yesterday, I was in a really bad car accident in New York City. In fact, my car is totaled. I've been studying EFT for a few months and had just completed the Level 2 and Level 3 workshops, so, faced with the shock of being in an accident and not really sure what happened, I began tapping. Right away I was interrupted by helpful witness/ bystanders who opened my car door and proceeded to check me out and tell me not to move and that an ambulance and the police were coming. I ached all over but I could move all my parts and the only blood was from where the seatbelt scraped my neck and where I bit my tongue.

Before I could begin tapping in earnest, the ambulance arrived and the paramedics used the standard things like a collar and back board, even though I knew I didn't need them and said so. Getting me from the car using the back board and the collar really hurt, partly because I am not a skinny woman and in part because the way they did it really hurt my bruises!

As soon as I was in the ambulance and lashed to the board and gurney, I began tapping about my aches and shock and the trauma of the car hitting the metal stanchion of the overhead subway. I knew that the paramedics who were writing up stuff would think I needed psychiatric help if they heard me doing setups so I said the Setup Phrases in my head and physically tapped on the Karate Chop point, and then the crown chakra on the top of my head, the third eye, the face points, the collarbone, the underarm, and the abdomen rib points. When that didn't seem enough I tapped on the finger points.

I tapped for my guilt about totaling the car and said I forgive myself even though I still really wasn't sure what happened. I tapped for the driver of the other car, who claimed I hit him, and I forgave him because I didn't know whether he was right or wrong and at that point it didn't matter. I can't remember all the setup statements I used because I tapped on everything I could think of, including my son's reaction to the loss of the car and my daughter's reaction to the fact that she now had no car to use. I even did a mental movie and saw myself hitting the pole and being unable to move out of the way. I wasn't tired, but each round of tapping produced yawns, so I knew something was happening. In the hospital they put an IV needle in my arm in case it was needed, so imagine, if you will, tapping one-handed because of being lashed to a board, attached to a collar to prevent you from moving your neck, with tape over your forehead to keep you still on the gurney, and with an IV needle in your arm.

At the hospital it was hurry up and wait because I wasn't logged in right away, so I kept tapping about my bruises, aches and pains, how awful the board was, the pain in my head from being on the board, and the bruise at the Gamut point that was black and swollen but not painful. I tapped for my swollen and bleeding tongue and how it hurt to swallow around the lump in my throat. I even did one 9 Gamut round just to be on the safe side.

My husband arrived at the hospital about 11:30 AM and, seeing me tapping, didn't interrupt. He stayed with me and I continued to tap saying the set-ups mentally. Occasionally we talked and then I'd go back to tapping. After maybe another hour I finally saw a doctor and I was still tapping. I told him I was doing EFT. He had never heard of it and I wasn't really up to explaining, so I made a mental note to send him some information about it later.

I still have some aches and pains from injured muscles and I've been tapping on them, individually and compositely. I have a thermopedic mattress topper so I was able to sleep comfortably even before I managed to remove all the pain aspects. I did take some Tylenol but it was the tapping that made the difference. I wasn't able to breathe deeply due to a rib bruise but I kept tapping and finally got some relief after thinking about the pain being like a strap around my chest. In fact, I pictured a thick brown belt with a silver buckle that I was opening so I could throw the belt away. Finally, when I was lying down, the tightness eased and I was able to breathe deeper. Of course when I got up many of the aches came back, but anyone could see that the healing was proceeding faster than usual.

All in all, I feel incredibly fortunate to have survived the accident—and even more fortunate to have a tool like EFT to work with any time, anywhere, even under adverse conditions. Oh, and my husband has become a believer, too.

* * *

8

The Search
for Core Issues

Sometimes back pain is part of a larger problem, a symptom of a deeper, more important underlying situation. By far the fastest way to resolve a complex issue or clear up pain that resists treatment is to discover its *core issue*. Core issues are fundamental emotional imbalances, usually related to traumatic events.

There are many ways to approach core issues. In some cases they are obvious to the person in pain. When asked about when the pain started or what might be contributing to it, the reply is immediate. "I'll bet it has something to do with my husband's heart attack last fall." "My back hurts whenever I think about my wife's affair." "My back has been killing me ever since my business failed."

But most of the time, core issues are hidden from view. This is because the subconscious mind is a clever protector of secrets, including those that we hide from ourselves.

In some cases, our subconscious minds hide secrets that are truly awful. But when revealed to the light of day, most of our personal secrets don't amount to much.

The reason Tom can't give a presentation at work is because his fourth grade teacher embarrassed him in front of the class. The reason Ann can't lose weight is because when she was eight years old, her mother told her she would always be too fat to wear a swim suit. The reason John can't propose to Marie is because his older sister always told him that he was such a loser, no one would ever marry him.

As long as they hold an emotional charge, these secrets are powerful enough to shape a person's life — but as soon as they are uncovered and neutralized with EFT, core issues like these lose their power and become insignificant old memories.

This aspect of EFT never ceases to amaze me. Again and again I've worked with people while they dealt with incredibly painful memories, memories that controlled their lives and dictated where they would live, what career they would follow, what friends they would have, and everything else. Suddenly, after a few rounds of EFT tapping, they are completely transformed and no longer frightened, anxious, or afraid of old events. Instead, they're able to describe them as easily as if they were talking about the weather. As soon as old events and old memories lose their emotional charge, they lose their place of power in the subconscious mind.

Core Issue Questions

Two of the tools we use to find core issues are questions and fill-in-the-blank statements, such as:

What does this back pain remind me of?

When was the first time I felt this same pain?

If there is a deeper emotion underlying this pain, what might it be?

If this back pain were a book or a movie, what would its title be?

If it were a Broadway play, what would its plot be?

If I set this back pain to music, what would it be and why—a country song, hard rock, a symphony, a melancholy Argentine tango, a John Philip Sousa march?

Who or what is the pain in my back?

If I could live my life over again, what person or event would I prefer to skip?

When I relax and let my mind drift, I realize that this pain might have something to do with _____.

When I think about the pain in my back, I realize _____.

The worst mistake I ever made was to _____.

I have this big red ball of rage in my back, and it's all because _____…

Sometimes the questions aren't necessary because you intuitively know what the core issue is. But core issues are often clever about hiding, so being a good detective is an EFT asset.

If you can't think of anything, you can use EFT to ask your subconscious mind for assistance by tapping while you say:

Even though I can't think of anything right now, I'll let my clever subconscious mind answer these questions with answers that help.

Even though I have no idea where this pain came from or what words to use to find the cause, I choose to effortlessly and effectively allow my brilliant subconscious mind to uncover the core issue and bring the most effective thoughts, ideas, and words to my conscious mind for best results.

Even though my mind is a blank, my brilliant subconscious mind knows what to do to help this technique work.

Sometimes mentioning specific emotions will help trigger a memory. Try tapping while you say:

Even though I might have anger, sadness, guilt, sorrow, hurt, frustration, or other emotions that I can't identify, and they're here under the surface, I love and accept myself, I bless and forgive myself, and even though those feelings are hidden for now, I choose to welcome them as they emerge, knowing that it's safe to invite them into my conscious mind because with the help of EFT tapping, I can be safe in every way, no matter what.

Even though I may have anger in my back, I deeply and completely accept myself…

Even though I can't come up with specific emotions or past events, the truth is that when I think about betrayal, I clearly remember _____.

...when I think about feeling lost and helpless...

...when I think about feeling overwhelmed and confused...

...when I think about that crushing blow of disappointment, as though the floor had fallen out from under me, I remember how my peripheral vision closed in, as though I was in a dark tunnel, and my heart stopped....

You can turn any problem statement into an EFT Setup Phrase. For example:

Even though my lower back hurts and it's probably because I'm so worried about money, I choose to replace thoughts of lack with thoughts of abundance. Now my mantra is, "All my needs are taken care of."

Even though my middle back hurts, and I just want the world to get off my back, I would like to let go of all the guilt in my back and dwell on the thought that I have released the past and move forward with love in my heart.

Even though my upper back hurts just the way my heart hurts because no one loves me the way I want to be loved, I choose to affirm that life supports and loves me and I love and approve of myself.

If you're still not able to come up with an event, memory, or connection, no problem. Just make something up. As I often say, a made-up example can work even better than an actual event or memory.

As soon as you have something, real or imaginary, that's connected in any way to your pain, create a short or long Setup Phrase around it and begin tapping.

EFT can enhance any type of treatment or therapy, which is why so many chiropractors, physical therapists, massage therapists, physicians, personal trainers, nurses, and other health care practitioners incorporate tapping into their professional work. Here are two interesting reports from Roseanna Ellis, who has been using EFT with chronic pain clients for over three years. Roseanna is a licensed massage practitioner and physical therapist assistant.

Core Issues Release Severe Back Pain

by Roseanna Ellis

On a Friday night in the summer of 2006, I received a call from a woman begging me to come to her home because she had severe back pain. She said, "I threw my back out and I won't be able to see my doctor until Monday. Please come now."

When I arrived, Mary could barely walk. I treated her in the living room because she was unable to climb the stairs.

I tried all the therapy tricks I knew for about half an hour to no avail. Then I asked her, "What was happening when you first threw your back out?"

She said, "I was watching my daughter try on her wedding dress." Then she talked about the stress of the wedding and how everything was going wrong. We tapped for the stress, for everything going wrong, and how I can't take it, I can't rely on anyone.

The pain decreased from a 10 to a 4 She was able to get on and off my treatment table with slight discomfort, but she was very restricted in range of motion.

I asked her, "Why would your body be afraid to move?"

She answered, "I am a control freak and the wedding planner is not doing things my way and it is freaking me out."

We tapped for

Even though I am a control freak, I choose to believe that others can also be awesome at what they do. Even though I am a control freak, I choose to give this wedding planner an opportunity to help me. Even though this control freak attitude is causing this immense pain and robbing me of the joy of my daughter's wedding dreams, I choose to get over this nasty habit.

This helped her a lot. She was able to move her body in every direction with a pain level that had fallen to one I asked her what was keeping the pain at a one. She answered, "It is very hard for me to give up control."

We tapped for:

Even though I am making this wedding all about me and not my daughter, I deeply love myself and my daughter.

That did the trick. She sat up with a shocked look on her face and said, "You're right, it is more about me than my daughter." With that she exclaimed that the pain was a zero, jumped off the table, and gave me a great big hug.

I went over the next morning to give her a good stretch. She was still completely free from pain.

In another case, a 50-year-old man came to see me complaining of low back pain that was so intense, it measured a 10 on the 0-to-10 scale. He had very limited range of motion and could not bend over or twist without being in agony.

He was afraid that he would not be able to heal and would have to give up his golf, which he loved so much. He also feared getting old and becoming helpless.

We performed EFT for the issues of being bent over, being afraid of getting old, being afraid to move because of pain, and fearing that he would have to give up golf, his favorite sport.

Within about fifteen minutes his range of motion had improved and his pain decreased to seven. Then he began to speak about his stress at work. We tapped for his stress until his intensity fell to a zero for stress. His pain fell to zero and he began to move more easily. We tapped before every motion he performed until all motion was normal and he could twist and bend without pain. In fact, he was able to bend enough to touch the floor. Needless to say, he was very pleased with his session.

※ ※ ※

Our aches and pains can be attached to all kinds of past events, and often you won't realize until you start tapping what memories might be involved. In many cases the calendar plays a role, subconsciously reminding us of unhappy past events. In this next example, Nancy Privett works with a woman whose severe shoulder pain is connected to a painful anniversary.

Shoulder Pain and a Painful Anniversary

by Nancy Privett

Marie came to see me to use EFT for her sore left shoulder and upper arm. This area had been hurting for a few days. The muscles all around the shoulder were sore, as well as the ones going up into her neck and down into her upper arm. She had limited mobility and could not reach behind her to fasten her bra.

I asked Marie what had been going on around the time when she noticed the sore muscles and the only thing that came to her mind was that a few days previously she had been to New York City to see a show with friends and had been holding her purse tightly against her left side with her arm. The next day she woke up with the soreness.

I noticed that when Marie mentioned her problem she said: "I feel like my mother, all crippled up and can't move." When I asked about that, she said that her mother, who had died eight years previously and who had lived with Marie and her family for the last several years of her life, had a lot of physical problems, including arthritis in her shoulders.

Marie repeated the phrase about feeling like her mother several times when talking about her shoulder, which was a clue that the physical symptoms might be connected emotionally with something to do with her relationship with her mother. However, we began tapping on the physical limitations and pain, and right away Marie felt a difference. She went from a discomfort level of 8 on a scale of 0-to-10 to about a 5 out of 10. Some phrases we used were:

Even though I have this soreness in my shoulder…

Even though I can't move my arm the way I want to…

Even though I have this pain in my upper arm…

Even though it hurts to raise my arm…

Even though I can't reach behind my back…

Even though this pain goes up into my neck…

Even though it hurts more now in my neck than in my shoulder…

The discomfort was staying at a 5, so I decided to use something I learned from a previous EFT newsletter article based on NLP languaging. I have had good results with this technique before.

I asked Marie to focus on the discomfort and answer the following as quickly as possible: What color is the discomfort? Is it bigger or smaller than your hand? Is it transparent or solid? Is it moving or still? And, most importantly: If it were associated with a feeling, what would that be?

To Marie's surprise, the answer to the last question was "sadness." So we tapped on that:

Even though I have this sadness in my shoulder...

Before we had completed the round of tapping, she said, "Oh! Of course!" She then told me that the eighth anniversary of her mother's death was in three days, and she was going to be away on a business trip on that day. She began crying, saying that she didn't realize how important it was to be home on that day. (Her mother had died suddenly and unexpectedly at home, in Marie's arms.) We then tapped on:

Even though I am very sad that I won't be home on the anniversary of mom's death...

When that round ended, Marie said that she had always felt bad about the event of her mother's death because, even though her mother had died in her arms, Marie felt like she hadn't said the right things to her as she was passing in order to comfort her. We tapped on:

Even though I feel guilty and bad that I didn't give mom the comfort she needed as she was dying in my arms...

Even though I didn't say the right thing to her as she died in my arms...

Even though I should have known the right thing to say to comfort mom as she was dying in my arms...

Notice the reference to the fact that Marie's mother had died in Marie's arms, and it was her shoulder and upper arm that was now hurting.

I then suggested to Marie that it really was a lovely and comforting thing in itself that her mother died in her daughter's arms. I said, "Just think, when you die, wouldn't it be nice to be in held in one of your children's arms when it happened?" She said she hadn't thought of that, but it was true.

The session was ending and Marie's shoulder discomfort was still a 5 on a scale of 0-to-10, but she said that "everything feels different." I had an intuitive feeling that after sleeping, her balance would be restored in the morning.

The next morning she called to say that she felt great and that all her shoulder and arm and neck pain was completely gone. She also felt lighter about her mother's death and didn't feel the sadness that she wouldn't be home for the anniversary. EFT resolved both the physical symptoms and the underlying emotional cause.

❊ ❊ ❊

Bypassing Core Issues

For the record, it's possible to treat back pain with simple Setup Phrases that acknowledge core issues without specifically addressing them. For example:

Even though I don't know where this pain came from, it doesn't matter how it started because my body is already, at a deep level, repairing itself, fixing my energy flow, and correcting whatever underlying causes contribute to the pain.

Even though there may be underlying emotional causes for this pain in my back, and my conscious mind doesn't know what they are, it doesn't matter because my subconscious mind is already removing the emotional charge that connects me to events and memories that helped trigger this pain.

Even though I've been trying without success to find the core issues that created this pain in my back, I fully and completely accept myself, and I realize that I may never know what the causes are, and that's okay because my mind and body are already removing the emotional causes, performing subconscious surgery, releasing energy blocks and the pain that they cause.

Even though I feel disappointed and frustrated because I can't figure out where this pain in my back came from or why it had to be there, it truly doesn't matter because I choose to let go of this pain and release it safely and effectively, just by balancing my body's energy.

Even though my conscious mind isn't able to make sense of this pain in my back, I fully and completely accept myself, I love and forgive myself and my back, and I rejoice that my body knows exactly what to do to release this pain and let it go.

Sneaking Up on the Core Issue

Sometimes the emotional reason for back pain is an issue so overwhelming that it seems beyond help. It's the "Big One" that the person doesn't want to touch. It may be a major form of guilt they don't want to face or a trauma they don't want to revisit. Whatever it is, they "don't want to go there" and often won't even mention it to their therapist for fear the therapist will try to drag them through it.

Often they learn to dull the pain or sweep it under the rug. But it seethes under the surface anyway, influencing their thoughts, their responses and their everyday lives. It represents pain. It's like walking on thorns. They would rather retain their less-than-truly-functional lives than come face to face with this issue. Their lives will get better, they hope, if they just address life's minor irritations and leave the "Big One" alone.

Fortunately, we have a method with EFT whereby we can tip-toe up to the issue, circle around it, take the edge off and gradually spiral in closer until that festering boil is skillfully lanced. All this with minimal pain. The concept is simple but it may take some practice before the practitioner can claim mastery.

It starts with a very general approach. I suggest asking clients to simply say...

The Big One

and then rank their 0-to-10 intensity regarding the mere mention of the issue. They also rank their pain and other physical symptoms, such as a pounding heart, sweating, constricted throat, etc. We then use EFT in a general way to help take the edge off.

>*Even though I have discomfort about this issue…*
>
>*Even though this thing seems too big for me…*
>
>*Even though just thinking about it bothers me…*
>
>*Even though my heart is pounding…*
>
>*Even though (other physical symptoms)…*

The details of the issue are ignored for now because the main purpose here is to minimize pain by taking the edge off. We are purposely sneaking up on the problem with gentleness as our goal. Do several rounds of EFT in this more general way until you see or experience signs of relaxation. That tell-tale "sigh" that I point out in our videotapes is a good clue. Then I ask them to say again

>*The Big One*

and re-rank their 0-to-10 intensities on this statement. Chances are the emotional responses will be lower and the physical symptoms will likely be down as well. I keep repeating this procedure until it seems appropriate to ask…

>*Is there any part of this issue that you could talk about comfortably?*

This simple procedure often opens the door, making it possible for the person to acknowledge or describe at least part of the issue. From there, it is simply a matter of getting more and more detailed. Take some of the edge off, get more detailed. Take some of the edge off, get more detailed. Take some of the edge off, get more detailed.

The client may experience some emotional discomfort in the process. After all, this *is* the "Big One." But, in my experience, it is much less than it might have been *and* this is probably the last time they will have any such discomfort (if they have any at all). Assuming our usual degree of success, they can now walk on velvet instead of thorns.

9

Eliminating
Self-sabotage

In any new project there are several ways in which we can interfere with our own progress. By becoming familiar with these ways, you can recognize them when they appear and then use EFT tapping to remove them.

By far the easiest way to reach a goal is with the cooperation of your subconscious mind. If there's agreement or congruence between what your conscious mind wants and what your subconscious mind has been programmed to accept as possible, everything is likely to flow smoothly toward the goal. But if there's disagreement or incongruence, the conscious mind doesn't have a chance. In that situation, the subconscious mind always wins. Somehow circumstances will conspire to prevent you from reaching your goal, and the conscious mind will probably never understand what happened or why. It will simply forget about the project or attribute your failure to bad luck or circumstances. It won't know that you yourself went out of your way to prevent your own success.

If you have ever made a New Year's resolution regarding your health or physical fitness, you may understand this syndrome all too well. Your conscious mind really wants to get your body into shape and enjoy the benefits of physical fitness, and you may even start your new exercise program with enthusiasm. But a week later, you're back on the sofa watching TV and eating potato chips.

If your back hurts, a vigorous exercise plan is probably the last thing from your mind, but it's a goal worth setting because the muscles that support your back, sides, and trunk work together to keep your back strong, flexible, and free from pain. As soon as you can, start walking, stretching, lifting weights, and doing exercises that build strength and stamina.

In addition, the combination of vigorous exercise and EFT is mutually reinforcing—exercise and the lymph circulation it stimulates help make EFT more effective, and EFT helps improve the positive effects of physical exercise.

Still, understanding this intellectually and embracing it emotionally are two different concepts. Do you resist exercising for reasons that have nothing to do with muscle spasms and pain? Sometimes the reasons for resisting are deeper than you think. Here Dr. Carol Solomon shows us how to get to these deeper issues and collapse them with EFT.

Using EFT to Overcome the Resistance to Exercise

by Dr. Carol Solomon

My clients often develop resistance to exercise. They want to exercise, but either they don't feel motivated or don't enjoy it. They know they "should" exercise, but it can easily turn into an internal power struggle.

There can be other obstacles to overcome as well. Some women feel too embarrassed, ashamed and/or self-conscious to go the gym at their current weight. So they avoid the activity that could actually help them lose weight. Others have perfectionist qualities; they think it won't make a difference, or it's not "worth it" unless they have time for a full 60-minute workout. So they don't go at all.

My client Susan wanted to talk about her resistance to going to the gym. She started out saying, "I love it...and I know I should do it, but it's not part of my routine...I need to make a plan." My intuition told me there was something deeper. I said, "Susan, it's not about planning." She said, "Why should I get excited or feel positive about anything? You know the other shoe is going to drop."

Two years ago, Susan's husband died while undergoing a routine sinus surgery. She pulled her life together and even began a new relationship. One week before this session, her new beau was diagnosed with colon cancer. It was no wonder that Susan felt as she did.

Even though I don't want to get excited about anything because I know the other shoe is going to drop...

Even though nothing turns out right for me, I choose to move forward anyway.

Even though everything always gets messed up...

Eyebrow: *Why should I get excited?*

Side of Eye: *I know the other shoe is going to drop...*

Under the Eye: *Things never turn out right for me...*

Under the Nose: *Why bother?*

Chin: *I feel cursed...*

Collarbone: *It's not fair...*

Under the Arm: *I've tried so hard...*

Top of Head: *Everything always gets messed up...*

Susan was also worried that she wouldn't keep up her momentum. In the two years since her husband's death, she had one crisis after another and couldn't follow through in her usual manner. Several attempts to make changes in her career got derailed when multiple crises occurred.

Even though I'm afraid I'll lose my momentum again... Even though I'm afraid I won't be able to maintain it... Even though I'm afraid something will happen, I choose to move forward anyway.

Eyebrow: *I've tried so hard.*

Side of Eye: *Everything's a crisis.*

Under the Eye: *I'm afraid something will happen.*

Under the Nose: *I'll just lose momentum again.*

Chin: *I won't be able to maintain it.*

Collarbone: *I'm not going to do it.*

Under the Arm: *You can't make me.*

Top of Head: *I don't want to be disappointed again.*

Eyebrow: *I choose to release these fears.*

Side of Eye: *I choose to move forward.*

Under the Eye: *I choose peace.*

Under the Nose: *I choose happiness.*

Chin: *I choose serenity.*

Collarbone: *I am grateful for all of the opportunities in my life.*

Under the Arm: *I choose to let it be fun and easy.*

Top of Head: *I can handle whatever comes.*

Since that session, which consisted of only two rounds of EFT, Susan began exercising with ease every day. She has also started a website and moved forward with significant changes in her career.

❊ ❊ ❊

Conditions That Interfere

Now let's consider some of the conditions that can interfere with your ability to reach the goals that you set, all of which can be addressed with EFT.

Psychological Reversal

The first obstacle that can interfere with your reaching a goal—such as the complete and total elimination of back pain—is your energy flow. If your energy is flowing in the right direction without obstacles or blockages, you're on your way. If your energy is blocked or reversed, the problem we call *psychological reversal* or *polarity reversal* interferes.

Tapping on the Karate Chop point or massaging the Sore Spot corrects this problem and gets the energy flowing as it should. It's possible to test for psychological reversal with muscle testing (kinesiology), but we save time by assuming that we might be psychologically reversed—it's a state that we all move in and out of several times a day—and correct the reversal before we start tapping. Thus, your Setup Phrase performs two vital functions: it focuses your mind on the problem you want to address, and it corrects psychological reversal if it happens to be in effect.

Self-talk and the Writings on Your Walls

The second potential stumbling block is your subconscious mind and its programming, which is reflected by your *self-talk*, the thoughts and statements that rattle around in your head at all hours of the day and night that have anything to do with you.

I call your self-talk's programming the *writings on your walls*. This writing contains all of the "rules" you grew up with—statements you heard as a child, reflecting your family or cultural conditioning, and ideas or notions, especially about yourself, that you've absorbed throughout your life.

It's hereditary. Back pain runs in my family.

The doctor looked at my X-rays and said I'll never stop hurting. He's a doctor, he must be right.

Everyone is used to me this way. This is how I'm supposed to be.

I'll never get any better. I've been disappointed too many times. Nothing works for me.

My job is here at home taking care of everyone. That's just how it is.

My job is running a business to support my family. That's what I'm supposed to do.

Tail-enders

Closely related to the writings on our walls are the *tail-enders* they inspire. Tail-enders are the "yes, but" statements that pop up when we try to set new goals or write new affirmations.

The most obvious tail-enders are the words we hear in our minds when we try out a new idea. These words often have a sarcastic ring to them: *Yeah, right. When pigs fly. I'll believe that when I see it. You must be kidding. Forget it. No way. Impossible.*

They are the nemesis of affirmations. A standard piece of advice in metaphysical circles is to turn negative self-talk around by stating the opposite. For example, if you hear yourself saying, "This is going to be a terrible day," try switching that to, "This is going to be a wonderful day." If your conscious and subconscious minds accept the affirmation, it probably will be a wonderful day—but what if they don't? That's when tail-enders create mischief.

Tail-enders can show up at the end of a "choices" statement, where you describe your goal, such as in this example:

> *Even though this back pain is killing me, I choose to be completely free from pain and enjoy full range of motion...*
>
> *...but I know that's never going to happen.*
>
> *...but I really don't deserve to be well.*
>
> *...but if I get well, I'm afraid my husband won't be as attentive and considerate as he is when I'm in pain.*
>
> *...I'll have to go back to the job I hate.*
>
> *...my daughter will be upset.*

Secondary Gain

Many **tail-enders** reflect a problem called secondary gain. Secondary gain is a psychiatric term meaning that the person has a hidden or unconscious reason for holding onto an undesirable condition.

The term applies to chronic pain cases in which the patient will lose certain benefits if he or she gets well, such as attention from others, monetary compensation for disability, or the ability to keep denying the original cause of the pain.

In metaphysics, the term "secondary gain" helps explain why we seem to run into barriers when it comes to manifesting our good. This occurs when we put a great deal of energy into visualizing, affirming, and treating for a new level of good and it either doesn't happen or the situation actually gets worse. The subconscious mind feels more secure in the disadvantaged state than going for improvement.

So your conscious mind might be saying:

I sincerely want to get over this problem…

while your subconscious mind says:

I don't want to get over this problem because…

I can't ever get over this problem because…

It would be dangerous for me to get over this problem…

I can't afford to get over this problem…

What benefits do you receive from your back pain? Does keeping the pain feel safe? Does releasing it feel dangerous? Does keeping the pain generate sympathy from others that you won't receive if you're well? Does keeping the pain allow you to avoid unpleasant situations? Does keeping the pain give you financial rewards that you won't receive if you get well? Do you feel you don't deserve to be well? Do you fear that if you get well, something bad will happen?

I don't want to give up my back pain because…

> *...if I get completely well, I'll lose my disability payments and I'll have to get a job, and who knows how long that will take, and I've been unemployed for so long that I wouldn't know where to go or what to do, and the whole idea is just too stressful...*

> *...if I get completely well, I'll have to move...*

> *...my back pain is such an important part of my identity that I won't know who I'll be if it goes away...*

> *...it's just too difficult...*

Some short, effective Setup Phrases that help neutralize the benefits of secondary gain include:

> *Even though I prefer to keep my back pain because _____, I deeply and completely accept myself anyway...*

> *Even though part of me wants to stay sick, disabled, and incapacitated, I fully and completely accept myself...*

> *Even though I like having this problem and intend to keep it and no one can make me give it up, so there, I nevertheless love and accept myself, I forgive and bless myself, I forgive my back, I forgive the part of me that keeps holding onto it, and I choose to facilitate the rapid healing of my back and all my emotions by releasing all my energy blocks beginning right now...*

A comprehensive Setup Phrase can deal with all of these stumbling blocks—psychological reversal, writings on your walls, tail-enders, and secondary gain issues—allowing you to reach your new goal with the full cooperation of your subconscious mind. Because it's important to release fears of not being able to cope or of being in danger if you let go of the pain, these Setup Phrases can include safety nets, reassurances that your brilliant subconscious mind can and will put you in the right place at the right time to bring benefits, not loss, into your life as you release the pain.

Even though I don't deserve to be completely well and free from pain, and I don't even want to get well, and I certainly don't deserve to get well, I choose to enthusiastically and creatively release all the guilt I used to feel about mistakes I made in the past…

Even though my back pain support group (or my friend Jane or my mom or my husband) will be upset if I get completely well and don't need their help any more, I choose to enjoy my own excellent health and my own independent, happy life knowing that they will adjust and adapt just fine…

Even though if I get completely well, I won't be eligible for disability payments any more, I welcome my perfect new job, which comes to me easily, comfortably, and with only good results.

Even though I have been receiving benefits from this back pain for a long time, I fully and completely accept myself. Even though I keep getting rewards for maintaining this back pain, I love and forgive myself. Even though this back pain prevents me from accomplishing my goals, and even though I may never let go of this back pain, I fully and completely accept myself, I love and forgive myself, I forgive my back, and I choose to be pleasantly surprised at how easy it is to instruct my subconscious mind to remove my attachment to any and all of the benefits and rewards that I receive or derive from maintaining this pain. I choose instead to receive rewards and benefits from releasing all of the pain in my back, opening myself to a new direction, and enjoying a new way of thinking and living. I choose to think and live in harmony with my goal of living a pain-free life beginning right now…

Of course, these statements are magnets for tail-enders, writings on your walls, and other psychological interference, but all of these can be treated with EFT. Just notice what comes into your mind and keep tapping.

Saying Goodbye to the Past

Another way to release core issues that are related to past events and contribute to self-sabotage is to tap while saying,

Even though _____ happened, it doesn't have to cause pain in my back any more. Even though _____ happened and I can't change the past, I can change my emotional connection to the past. Even though _____ happened, it doesn't affect me any more, I can relax about it and let it go.

10

Improving Results

In some cases, EFT may be working very well without your realizing it. In others, success may follow a simple change of strategy. This chapter explores some common reactions and provides suggestions for dealing with them.

Chasing the Pain

One result that often confuses those new to EFT is that with each round of tapping, their pain may find a new location, going from lower back to shoulder, from shoulder to neck, from neck to knee, and so on.

I believe that this moving pain is evidence of changing emotional issues and a clue that at least one core issue is working its way toward the surface. As you relieve each pain with EFT tapping, you relieve the emotional issues behind it. Staying with the pain and tapping through all of its manifestations usually causes its gradual reduction and elimination, especially if you stop along the way to tap on any emotionally charged memories that come to mind.

An example of chasing the pain might be:

Even though I have this sharp pointy arrow-like pain in my lower back...

Even though the pain in my lower back has disappeared, I now have a throbbing hot orange ball of pain at the base of my neck...

Even though I now have this small hard shiny black box of pain in my right hip...

Even though I now have this dull aching pain in my right thigh...

Even though I now have this sharp pointy red pain in my right knee...

Approach each of these new locations as though it is a new pain with a new Setup Phrase and tapping sequence.

In the next report, Marie LaForce, a registered nurse, describes how her client's pain moved from one location to another. This is a good example of how EFT's Basic Recipe did a thorough job of relieving pain. Because the pain eventually came back, I think that exploring emotional issues that may be contributing to the pain and, for that matter, the overall condition (spinal stenosis) would be of further value.

Chasing Spinal Stenosis Pain

by Marie LaForce

I saw a woman who was in pain for the entire summer and wasn't sure why. This fall she was diagnosed with spinal stenosis, a narrowing of the spinal column that was putting pressure on her nerves. She had been seeing a physical therapist for about three weeks and was not getting much relief from her pain. I asked her if she'd like to try EFT. She said, *"Why not?"*

We focused on the physical symptoms and began with her rubbing on the sore spot.

Even though I have this pain in my left butt cheek, I deeply and completely accept myself.

We followed the pain as it seemed most predominant (where she noticed it).

Even though I have this pain in my left hip...
Even though I have this pain in my left knee...
Even though I have this pain in my left thigh...
Even though I have this pain in my left hip...

The entire basic recipe was applied after each of the Setups with no shortcuts. After tapping on "my hip" for the second time, she reported that the pain was gone. She got up and moved. The pain was still gone. As she sat on the couch, she told me that she generally wasn't able to sit for that length of time without feeling very uncomfortable. She had no pain at all when I left.

I called her a month later. She said the pain stayed away for about a week and gradually started to reappear. When I talked to her she was quite uncomfortable again. I believe that continued tapping on the pain or other issues such as support (problems with the spine), etc., would have helped her to get at the additional aspects that were coming up.

* * *

Try Mental Tapping

Instead of tapping with your fingers, tap with your imagination. This requires focus and concentration, but when you tune out everything else and really feel the connection, this method works very well.

Try a little mental tapping every day. Its obvious advantages are that it can be done anywhere at any time, it's totally discreet, it won't disrupt anything, and no one will realize you're doing anything unusual.

Some who try this method visualize themselves tapping as though they're watching themselves in a mirror.

Another way to tap mentally is to picture a laser light shining straight onto your EFT points. The laser can be any color.

Still another approach is to imagine each EFT point pulsing or popping up on its own, like a button.

You can combine mental tapping with surrogate or proxy tapping to send balanced energy to others. As explained in the next section (Borrowing Benefits), this technique will help your back pain, too.

When you try mental tapping for the first time, do it in a quiet location with no distractions. With practice, you'll be able to tap in your mind with good results even in noisy environments.

Surrogate or Proxy Tapping

In surrogate or proxy tapping, you tap on something else—usually yourself or a photo—in place of the person you hope to help.

EFT practitioners do proxy tapping all the time when they tap in person or by phone with clients for their clients' problems. Students attending EFT workshops do it whenever they tap along with someone whose problem is being treated onstage. Anyone who taps along with our instructional DVDs does it, too. You will automatically do surrogate or proxy tapping whenever you work with a tapping buddy or with an EFT group.

Surrogate tapping can be used from any distance, from a few inches to thousands of miles. It can be done at any time, whenever you think of the person. You can tap on yourself for your own emotional responses at the same time, especially for emotions like worry, frustration, impatience, guilt, anger, fear, grief, or depression.

You can also do surrogate tapping to help animals, including family pets, animals in zoos or on farms, and wild animals.

There are three basic ways to proceed. You can:

Tap as though you are the person or animal you want to help,

> *Tap as though you are talking to the person or animal you want to help, or*

> *Tap as though you are describing the person or animal you want to help.*

For example, your friend Tom hurt his back playing baseball. If you're tapping with him in person, simply tap on yourself while saying his Setup Phrases along with him as both of you tap together:

> *Even though I hurt my back sliding into second base, I fully and completely accept myself. Even though I took a chance and it didn't pay off, I got tagged out and* ✓ *now my back is throbbing, I forgive and accept myself. Even though it was dumb to try stealing bases at my age, I did what I did and now I choose to release all this pain in my back...*

If you're by yourself and thinking about Tom, you can tap on yourself while using the same first-person Setup Phrase, above, or you can use a second-person Setup Phrase, as though you are talking to Tom:

> *Tom, even though you hurt your back sliding into second, I fully and completely accept you. Even though you took a chance that didn't pay off, you got tagged out and now your back is throbbing, you can forgive and accept yourself. Even though you're getting a little old to be stealing bases, the game is over, and now you can release all the pain in your back...*

Or you can use a third-person Setup Phrase, as though you're talking about Tom:

Even though Tom hurt his back sliding into second, I fully and completely accept him. Even though he took a chance that didn't pay off, he got tagged out and now his back is throbbing, he can forgive and accept himself. Even though he's getting a little old to be stealing bases, the game is over, and now he can release all the pain in his back…

Borrowing Benefits

Did you know that tapping on behalf of others can help clear your own back pain? This is one of the more unusual aspects of EFT, and it's one of the most exciting. Talk about a win-win situation. Every time you help someone else, you help yourself.

You can borrow benefits by tapping as you study this book, sending your energy to the people whose stories you're reading. You can borrow benefits by tapping as you watch our EFT seminars on DVD, or watch the news on television, or watch commercials for back pain remedies and anything else. You can tap on behalf of characters in books, plays, movies, magazines, and online reports. You can tap on behalf of your boss, co-workers, customers, friends, neighbors, children, spouse, parents, other relatives, and people you've never met. Whenever you practice sending balanced energy their way, you'll feel better yourself. And if they're real people with real problems, your energy will make a difference in their lives as well.

You can do this tapping in person, such as while showing your brother-in-law how to relieve his sciatica, or from a distance (using surrogate or proxy tapping), or by phone.

The Borrowing Benefits phenomenon is so powerful and fascinating that I conducted an entire seminar on this theme, and it's available on DVD. At the beginning of each section, I remind those watching to select a personal problem, focus on it for a moment, and then set it aside. While your conscious mind is busy tapping along with the seminar audience, your subconscious mind will include your own situation in every tapping session.

The benefits you receive, or "borrow," don't have to be related in any way to the situations you tap for. If your back is hurting, just focus for a moment on how it hurts, then give your undivided attention to the person you want to help. You can tap with a golfer to improve his swing, tap with a student to improve her grades, tap with a dieter about losing weight, or even tap for the family dog to help her indigestion—and all the while, your back will feel better.

In one EFT workshop, a man who owned a small business was stressed and distracted by a financial crisis that he didn't know how to resolve. He felt too overwhelmed to think straight. The instructor asked whether anyone in the group was in pain, and a woman asked for help with her menstrual cramps. Soon everyone in the room was tapping and saying, "Even though these cramps are killing me, I fully and completely accept myself…" Two minutes later the woman exclaimed that her cramps had completely disappeared—and the businessman excitedly announced, "While I was tapping about my menstrual cramps, I realized exactly how to fix my company's problem."

After introducing the "Borrowing Benefits" feature of EFT, I received many enthusiastic responses. For many, it represents a big step toward speed and efficiency in the delivery of these procedures.

The process also provides an additional measure of emotional safety. As you know, EFT is normally quite gentle but a few people tune in to some pretty intense stuff and it takes awhile to bring them down. With the Borrowing Benefits feature, however, clients merely identify their issues and then tap along with someone else on an issue that is seemingly quite different. Thus a sort of detachment is injected into the process while the original issues are being addressed "in the background." In this way it's like the Tearless Trauma Technique.

This way of defining and approaching problems, in my experience, helps to minimize any unwanted intensity while still getting the job done. The process may or may not give complete resolution to an issue but, properly done, it is likely to at least take the edge off, and probably much more. Very efficient. Very useful. Very humane.

Borrowing Benefits can also be a superb way to conveniently get at core issues so that truly deep work can be done. An easy way to tap along with creative EFT sessions is to pick certain from our EFT training videos, which are filled with actual sessions, many of which are quite involved. You can identify your own issue and then tap along with the video while in your living room.

Here's an example of this from Melissa Derasmo.

Borrowing Benefits from DVDs Eliminates Pain

by Melissa Derasmo

This is just a note to confirm yet again the enormous value of your DVDs. I had been struggling with a severe neck and shoulder pain (always hovering around a level of intensity of 8 out of 10) for the last six months and had been tapping for it for the last four months with little to no improvement. I was quite convinced that this sharp pain fell into the impossible-to-fix category—until I watched your session with Beth on the "From EFT to the Palace of Possibilities" DVD set.

As a habit, I tap along with every session on the DVDs, and this one was no exception. It appears that Beth's chronic pain was due in part to her issue of considering herself a savior—someone who needed to save everyone and fix the world. While this was not at all something I could identify with, I tapped along anyway. When the session was over, Beth's pain was gone—and so was mine!

This really shocked me. I had no idea that my wanting to fix everyone I met with EFT was in fact, my way of playing the savior. I did quite a few rounds on every aspect I could come up with on this subject and the pain has yet to reappear—and I'm quite sure that it won't.

So a major thank-you for this session you did with Beth. I was able to get such wonderful results just by tapping along!

❀ ❀ ❀

Last, here is a suggestion for Borrowing Benefits while watching television or movies from Dr. Carol Look. She writes, "I ask clients who watch a great deal of television or frequent movie theatres to tap for the characters' distress: 'Even though she feels insecure around that man...' 'Even though she won't admit the failure is her fault...' 'Even though he's afraid to confront the situation...' The clients do not have to identify their own issues first, just tap for the distress that their own system can't help but tune into as a result of witnessing someone else's discomfort on the big screen."

You can even tap for the people in back pain commercials.

This is a clever way of helping the subconscious mind neutralize some of the emotional charge connected to past events, making it easier to recognize, deal with, or simply release old problems. Tapping on behalf of fictional characters or real people you've never met brings you as many benefits as tapping on behalf of your best friend. Isn't that fascinating?

Additional Tapping Procedures

You may not ever need the floor-to-ceiling eye roll, the collarbone breathing exercise, or the 9 Gamut treatment, but take a minute to become familiar with them so that you'll have them in your repertoire of EFT procedures. These techniques are both subtle and powerful, and they can trigger a breakthrough when blocked energy refuses to move.

The Floor-to-ceiling Eye Roll

This is a useful short cut when you have brought the intensity of the problem down to a low level, such as a 1 or 2 on the 0-to-10 scale. It takes only six seconds to perform and, when successful, it will take you to zero without having to do another round of The Basic Recipe.

To perform it, simply repeat your Reminder Phrase while you tap the Gamut point continuously (hold your head steady) and take six seconds to slowly move your eyes from hard down to the floor to hard up to the ceiling.

Remember that this is an eye exercise, and your eyes are more likely to roll smoothly if they have something to follow. To achieve this result, hold both arms straight down in front of you. Keeping your head straight, lower your gaze to the floor. Begin tapping with one hand on the Gamut point of the other, and slowly raise both hands (keep your elbows straight) until they are straight out in front of you, then continue moving up until they are pointing straight at the ceiling.

At the beginning of this eye exercise, while you face straight ahead, you won't be able to see either hand. As you slowly swing your hands up, the fingertips of the tapped-on hand will move into view. Keep your eyes on the fingertips while your hand continues all the way up to the ceiling, at which point they will disappear again.

Reverse the direction and slowly bring your hands back down, tapping on the Gamut point all the while.

Collarbone Breathing

In a few cases, perhaps five percent, a unique form of energy disorganization occurs within the body that impedes the progress of EFT. Its details are well beyond the scope of this book but I *can* show you how to correct the problem. I call it the Collarbone Breathing Problem not because there is something wrong with anyone's collarbones or one's breathing. Rather, it is named for its correction, the collarbone breathing exercise. This correction was developed by Dr. Roger Callahan and need only be "thrown in" in cases where persistence with basic EFT is not showing results. It takes about two minutes to perform, and it may clear the way for the normal operation of otherwise impeded EFT procedures.

Collarbone Breathing Exercise

While you can start with either hand, I'm going to assume you are starting with the right hand. Keep your elbows and arms away from your body so that the only things touching it are your fingertips and knuckles. Most people tend to drop their elbows, so remind yourself throughout the exercise to keep your elbows up, parallel to the floor, not touching the torso.

Place two fingers of your right hand on your right collarbone point. With two fingers of your left hand (keep your right elbow up), tap the right hand's Gamut point continuously while you perform the following five breathing exercises:

Breathe half way in and hold it for seven taps.

Breathe all the way in and hold it for seven taps.

Breathe half way out and hold it for seven taps.

Breathe all the way out and hold it for seven taps.

Breathe normally for seven taps.

Place the two fingers of your right hand on your *left* collarbone point and, while continuously tapping the Gamut point, do the five breathing exercises.

Next, bend the fingers of your right hand so that the second joint or "knuckles" are prominent. Place these knuckles on your right collarbone point and tap the right hand's Gamut point continuously while doing the five breathing exercises.

Repeat this by placing the right knuckles on the left collarbone point.

You are now half way done. You complete the collarbone breathing exercise by repeating the entire procedure using the fingertips and knuckles of the *left* hand. You will be tapping the *left* Gamut point with the fingertips of the *right* hand.

If you have used EFT persistently and your results are either slow or non-existent, start each round of basic EFT with the collarbone breathing exercise. You may find that it "clears the way" and allows dramatic relief.

11

Pain, Anger, and Metaphors

By now you understand how EFT can be used to relieve back pain and every other kind of pain. In fact, at this point you know more than many EFT practitioners. You've gone far beyond mechanical EFT and are well on your way to EFT artistry.

At this point I'd like to return to Dr. Sarno's theory of back pain—that your back hurts because you're angry —and focus on using EFT as a tool for forgiving, forgetting, and letting go of anger.

Take another look at the words and phrases you use unconsciously and habitually.

Metaphors and Back Pain

Metaphors are colorful words or phrases that we use as analogies to describe things, people, and situations. They can be entertaining and expressive, but psychologists warn that our bodies take all of the words we use seriously.

> *She's such a pain in the neck.*

If you refer to someone in your life as a "pain in the neck" long enough or often enough, guess what—you can wind up with a pain in your neck.

That's why skilled EFT practitioners ask their pain clients questions like:

> *Who's stuck in your spine?*
>
> *Who is the pain in your neck?*
>
> *What's the heavy weight that you're carrying?*
>
> *Who stabbed you in the back?*

Think of what your body might do with some common expressions like:

> *My back is killing me.*
>
> *This pain is driving me crazy.*

It's always a good idea to pay attention to the images we use—and to be sure that our bodies aren't interpreting those images as instructions! The following report by Gary Clark demonstrates this principle well.

Clearing a Back Pain Metaphor

by Gary Clark

After watching the first three sets of EFT instruction DVDs, I decided to start using EFT in my practice. I am a Myotherapist so I deal mainly with people's muscle pain.

When a new patient arrived to have her back pain treated, I was surprised to find that she didn't have much in the way of the trigger points that usually cause this type of pain.

After dealing with the few soft-tissue problems I could find, her pain level fell from a 10 to an 8.

"Okay," I said , "can you point to the exact place where it hurts?"

She indicated the top of the sacrum. I placed my hand there and said, "If this part of your back could talk to you, what would it say?"

Quick as a flash she said, "Escape."

"And what do you want to escape from?"

"Work." she replied.

"And what is it about work that you want to escape from?"

"Oh," she said, "I run my own business, and work has been terribly slow lately. It's a real pain in the butt."

"Did you hear what you just said?" I asked.

"Oh my God," she exclaimed, "I've been telling everyone for the last three weeks that work is a pain in the butt."

I grinned and said, "Be careful what you wish for. You just might get it."

I quickly taught her EFT and we did two rounds of

Even though I have been saying that work is a pain in the butt, I truly and deeply accept myself...

Those two rounds completely cleared the pain. Later, I couldn't help thinking that I could have saved us both a lot of time if I had used EFT right away.

❈ ❈ ❈

Here is a fascinating report from EFT practitioner Dale Teplitz about how literal the mind can be when it generates pain.

Shooting Back Pain—an Amazing Metaphor

by Dale Teplitz

Metaphors often crop up while doing EFT. I find them of great value in providing clues to the cause of physical and emotional pain. Sorting through the metaphors and all their possible meanings is often well worth the effort. Metaphors can provide examples of how we literally "store" trauma and experiences in our body's energy system. The EFT practitioner can be of value by noticing the metaphor and taking the client in that direction. Here is a stunning example in which the client identified her own metaphor.

Betty attended a Level 2 EFT workshop that I taught in Los Angeles in March, 2006. When I asked whether anyone had a difficult physical symptom they would like to work on in front of the group, Betty volunteered. She had been trying to rid herself of low back pain for years. She suggested that it was a really tough one! Nothing she tried had worked. She was stumped about the relationship between this pain and any particular emotions.

As she bravely ascended the podium to work with me, Betty reported having a sharp pain that ran from her lower back to her right foot. Her doctor called it sciatica.

Betty is a very bright, articulate, and introspective woman in her sixties who has been a marriage and family therapist for over 20 years. She spent much of her adult life as a tireless seeker of healing for her own childhood wounds as well as those of her clients.

Her life was filled with struggles, which began at the moment of her own birth, a traumatic C-section. Many serious challenges involving family relationship issues followed.

When Betty was a vulnerable 14 years old, her father took his own life. At that moment, her childhood ended. She was forced to become the "parent" to her mother. Her young life was filled with burden.

In the workshop, we began tapping about her back pain with the basic EFT recipe. While tapping, I encouraged her to describe the pain in increasingly specific ways. When I asked how the pain moved, she reported that it "shot" from her lower back to the large toe of her right foot.

As she traced the pain with her hand to demonstrate to us where it was, her jaw dropped. In this "light bulb" moment, Betty remembered that when her father ended his life, he tied a shoelace from the big toe of his right foot to the trigger of the shotgun he used to shoot himself in the head. He was literally "shooting from the toe!"

All of us, including Betty, were astonished at the unfolding metaphor. By the look on her face, she had no doubt about the connection between the shooting pain to her toe and her father's death. Betty and I began to unravel the metaphor as we tapped each point.

This shooting pain. This shooting toe pain. Dad shooting himself in the head pain...

For every thought and memory she expressed, we tapped. Layers of deep trauma, shame, and grief welled up and were collapsed with EFT within minutes. They were gradually replaced with compassion for what she and her father had been through. The shooting pain disappeared. Betty looked lighter!

Eighteen months later, Betty reports that the shooting pain has not returned. Although now retired from counseling, Betty continues to use EFT as an important piece to the healing puzzle for herself, her family and friends.

❊ ❊ ❊

The next report illustrates how quickly a well-timed question can stop pain in its tracks. When Gillian Wightman's son complained of a stabbing pain between his shoulder blades, she asked him who stabbed him in the back. Great question!

She Stabbed Him in the Back

by Gillian Wightman

Two years ago my son, who was then 16, had an acute stabbing pain in his back. He resisted the idea of using EFT for the pain as he argued it was a physical problem that needed manipulation. My husband and I are trained in CranioSacral therapy so I knew I had the skills to treat him if this was the case. However, I also knew this pain had started when it became clear that things had changed between him and a girl he had had a crush on for years. They had not embarked on a relationship but had an understanding, and one night at a group event she treated him very badly. I think it was her clumsy way of letting him know her feelings had changed that hurt him so much. The pain appeared the next day.

When he came begging for help with his back, I got him to lie on the couch and put my hands under his back, where the pain was, right in between the shoulder blades. I asked him how the pain felt and he described it as if a knife was stabbing into his back. I waited a little and then asked,

So who stabbed you in the back?

He shouted out, ***"Becky!"*** Then he said, "Oh my, you got me didn't you? How do you do that?" He was laughing and he agreed to try EFT. We worked through all his feelings of frustration and confusion. She wouldn't talk to him and he had no idea what had happened or what he had done wrong. There were a lot of very painful emotions in his back. We started with

> *Even though Becky stabbed me in the back...*

and that immediately brought his pain from a 10 down to a 2 or 3. We then fine-tuned it by tapping for different aspects of his anger, hurt, and confusion. Tapping through all of his heartbreak totally relieved this acute pain and I am happy to say he now enjoys a good platonic relationship with this girl.

❖ ❖ ❖

Letting Go of Anger

If the healing process has one main theme, in my mind, it's forgiveness. EFT will work even if you hold onto grudges, but it works better if you let them go. After all, grudges and anger are negative emotions, and negative emotions occupy the same meridian energy blocks that cause pain.

Occasionally someone demonstrates just how powerful the connection is. Consider what happened to Caroline, who worked for many years as a school bus driver. Two years ago, her school van was rear-ended by a truck in an accident that left her with painful injuries.

Caroline attended an EFT training class seven months after the accident, not because she was interested in the subject but because she was delivering something for the instructor. As long as she was there, she decided to tap along with the group and she was soon startled to realize that over 70 percent of her chronic pain from the accident had spontaneously disappeared. "I can't believe it," she exclaimed. "This stuff works better than seven months of physical therapy!"

Soon the whole class was tapping with her, focusing on the accident, the school van, the pain, the seven months of physical therapy, and the frustration of being injured. Caroline kept feeling better and better. In fact, her pain completely disappeared—until the instructor had everyone say, "I completely forgive the man who rear-ended my van."

While the rest of the class continued tapping, Caroline froze. Her eyes grew wide with that deer-in-the-headlights look, she couldn't move, and as soon as the round was over, she complained, "Now the pain is worse than it was before."

Despite understanding that there was a clear connection between her unforgiveness and her pain, Caroline found it impossible to let go of her anger toward the other driver. As she told the class, "I can't forgive him. That's God's job. If God wants to forgive him, that's fine, but it's not my job."

With a great deal of coaxing, she was eventually able to say something far less threatening. She tapped and said,

Even though I can't forgive the guy who crashed into me, I would like to consider the possibility of perhaps one day, some day, maybe forgiving him just a little.

That was at least a tiny step in the right direction, but more than that she refused to consider.

Still, the message got through, and every day Caroline's body reminded her of the pain that unforgiveness can cause. A large black sun just to the right of her shoulder blade shot painful black rays into her back and shoulder, interfering with her sleep, exercise, and every other aspect of her life. Caroline understood intellectually that the pain was linked to her anger, and she tried through prayer and meditation to release it, but without success. When she became sufficiently desperate, she asked the EFT instructor for help.

Caroline was soon combining EFT with Dr. Carrington's one-percent solution (see page 266). She focused on her anger and frustration toward the man who was her boss at the time of the accident because he refused to call an ambulance, insisting that she didn't need medical attention. She drove herself to her own doctor, who believed her brain was bleeding and sent her to an emergency room where she was treated for multiple injuries.

At the time of the accident, while she waited at a red light behind other vehicles, Caroline had a split second before impact in which to turn the wheel so that her van didn't crash into the car in front of her. Instead of being applauded for preventing death or injury to others, she was blamed for causing the accident. Workman's compensation bureaucrats denied her claim while making false accusations and repeatedly misplacing her proof of injury.

Caroline had many legitimate grievances, but as she tapped, vented, and occasionally cried, her dark cloud of anger, frustration, and unforgiveness lifted, and she was soon saying, "It was just an accident. It's over. And thanks to being laid off, I went back to school, took classes that I would never have been able to take, completed my training as an Emergency Medical Technician, and am enrolled in a Ph.D. program. If it weren't for the accident, I would never have been able to do these things." Note the cognitive shift here. For almost two years, Caroline had repeated her story to anyone who would listen with the same words and the same story line. Suddenly her perspective shifted and she looked at it entirely differently.

By the end of her 20-minute session, Caroline was enthusiastically tapping to release not just one percent of her anger and unforgiveness, but rather all of it, and she was laughing, rejoicing, sighing, stretching, and thoroughly enjoying her new pain-free life. In the two months that followed, she reported ever-increasing freedom from pain, improved range of motion, and growing happiness and optimism.

In the early days of EFT, Adrienne Fowlie and I were giving a workshop for therapists. To test us, some of the therapists brought their "tough clients" for us to work with, one of whom was a middle-aged lady who had been in several automobile accidents two years prior. I remember her telling me that she had a metal plate in her neck and that her right arm was beset with pain that was *Always* at a 9 or 10. I mean *always*. It never let up.

We did two rounds of basic EFT on her arm pain with no result. Then I asked her,

If there was an emotional contributor to this pain, what would it be?

She didn't hesitate for even an instant and let loose an angry tirade about the driver of the car that hit her, the incompetence of her physicians, and on and on. There was nothing subtle about her anger. Her face took on a red complexion and the veins stood out in her neck. If she were a volcano, I would have evacuated the building.

We did two or three rounds—about two minutes total—of tapping on the anger and she quickly calmed down. She spoke of the incident in much calmer terms and the pain in her arm went to zero. Further, her therapist phoned Adrienne two months later and reported that the arm pain remained at a zero. It never came back.

Anger is one of those emotions that can help us or harm us. In fairness to anger, it can motivate us to act in order to change harmful situations, but most of the time it just festers or causes new problems. Fortunately, once we uncover anger, it's easy to treat and transform with EFT.

Here's a similar example from Dr. El March.

Severe Back Pain Subsides After Anger Issue Uncovered
by Dr. El March

I've been in the field of Orthomolecular Medicine for many years, so when Ed came to me for lower back pain after three months of not being able to go to work or move in any direction, we tried a number of things in an effort to get him up and running.

I sent him to chiropractors, had him do exercises, and put him on mega-vitamin therapy, only to have him return with severe pain every few months and later every few years. This year Ed came to my office completely stiff and in great pain, looking for more exercises and advice to ease the situation. This time I decided to try the EFT method on him and with his permission we started.

I knew that he had been suffering from this problem for more than ten years. I first did three rounds of basic EFT and tapped with him for the pain, which went from a 10 to 5 and back up to 10 again.

We started talking and I learned he had been laid off from his job couple of years back and is now in business for himself. His business is stressful and he cannot afford to take the time off.

So we tapped for:

Even though this pain is the only way that I can rest and spend some time at home without feeling guilty that I'm not making any income...

We also tapped on:

Even though I don't believe this method is going to do anything for me...

During these rounds of tapping the pain dropped to an 8 and then to a 5, but no matter how many more rounds we did, it stayed stuck, going back and forth between 5 and 8.

Then I asked Ed to explain his emotions toward the pain and he said, "Anger." He went on to tell me the story of how his back pain had come about.

I was employed at a financial institution as a senior computer center analyst. On the day this happened I was monitoring the progress on a job I had given one of my staff to do when some computers were delivered to our laboratory. As I was looking for someone to set the computers up, my manager, Dan, walked in and asked me to haul the computers to a different location in the lab where they were waiting for installation.

I felt his action was uncalled for and disrespectful to my seniority and grade level. This was completely out of line and not part of my functions, and I felt belittled in front of the employees who reported directly to me. As I was lifting one of the boxes, the muscle in my back made a noise and I felt heat rushing through my lower back. I couldn't move after that. I was sent home and stayed on short-term disability for about three months. I first came to see you one month before I went back to work.

After hearing this explanation, I decided to tap with Ed on the feelings he had going back to 1994 and his manager's actions:

Even though my manager was disrespectful to me and belittled me in front of my staff and I don't believe he had the right to ask me to do what he did, I completely and lovingly accept myself, I love and respect myself, I forgive myself and I forgive Dan.

Once we finished tapping on this the pain dropped from 8 to 3. Ed kept calling Dan an ass so I did another round of tapping on:

Even though Dan behaved like a complete ass and was completely out of line for asking me to move the computers, I completely and lovingly accept myself. I love and forgive myself and I forgive Dan.

Two rounds of EFT and Ed's pain was completely gone. He was amazed and did not believe it would last. I checked with him the next day, the next week, and again a few months later. The pain has still not returned.

I think EFT has added quite an edge to my regular practices. I have used it on myself and family members to quickly treat shoulder pain, headaches, nausea, and so on. This method is absolutely invaluable.

❊ ❊ ❊

Kaye Bewley in the U.K. describes how her client failed to achieve any relief for her long-held back pain from either the medical profession or alternative therapies. Note how Kaye handled the core issue, which her client did not want to express.

Anger and Rage Are at the Root of This Back Pain

by Kaye Bewley

When Alison arrived on my doorstep, her face was creased with a deep, furrowed frown. She had the look of someone who had been in pain for a long time and had come to accept it as a burden. Alison said she had been plagued with a pain in her upper back for about four years and pain in her lower back for the past 25 years.

Recently she had taken drugs for the pain and unfortunately reacted very badly to them. She even had to be admitted to the hospital's coronary ward because they thought she was having a heart attack. She said it felt as though a tight band had been drawn across her chest. Also, the weekend prior to seeing me, she had been doing some exercises and strained her shoulder so badly that she couldn't raise her arm.

She wondered whether EFT would be able to do something for her as she had already spent over £2,000 on alternative therapies that hadn't worked.

We sat down and concentrated on the pain in her back, which she rated at an 8. After one round it went down slightly to 7, so we completed another couple of rounds, one with negative statements such as,

I don't want to release this pain in my back...

and the next with positive statements such as,

I may consider releasing this pain in my back...
I can choose to be without this pain in my back...

After completing these rounds, she rated the pain as going down to a 5, and for the first time in a long time, she smiled.

Another few rounds concentrated on the pain in her back, after which we tentatively began to explore the emotional issues that might be behind it.

Alison mentioned that her social life was okay, but she admitted to having some problems at work, such as having to cover for everyone who had been off sick and feeling as though she couldn't let the company down. She had recently been verbally abused by a customer without any support from her boss, who witnessed the situation. She had also been given extra tasks which were beyond her physical capabilities. We went through another round of tapping on specific issues related to these instances, and finally came to the crux of her pain—anger.

She began to explore some problems she had been experiencing with a manipulative, inconsiderate step-brother. He had upset one of her friends with his cheating and lies, and she felt very hurt by that.

She said there were many scenes that gave rise to the angry feelings inside, but when I asked her to describe one, she said she didn't want to express it. This was okay, as with EFT the therapist doesn't need to know all the details of your emotional experiences, so we simply picked a word that related to the scene and concentrated on that.

Thus a "rage" rating of 8 was decided upon and we tapped on the EFT points. Three rounds of tapping brought her anger levels down from 8 to 7½…then to 5…then to 2.

Alison then mentioned a couple of long-standing issues that were coming into focus about her step-brother. She felt angry because he wasn't supportive towards her parents when they became ill. Her rage at him in that particular situation was higher than a 10, but after tapping for several rounds, we managed to bring it down to a 3, which was wonderful.

At this point we took a well-earned breather and I explained about how the words of others condition our thoughts. I gave a few examples, but none of them fit with her until I asked her if she had ever been told by her parents not to leave the table until she had finished her meal.

Aha! She said her mum always made her sit at the table and finish her vegetables and threatened her with not being able to have her pudding if she didn't eat all of her main meal.

She found the funny side of this as we tapped on it, using it as a metaphor for the way things kept happening in her life now. We found a pattern in that she always had to work hard before she was able to get any pleasure in life, but she ended up not getting any pleasure after all because she there was always something she had to do before she was able to relax.

Now she found herself working hard under the management of a boss who didn't stand up for her and under the direction of supervisor who made her do work she wasn't able to keep up with physically, on top of which she had to take care of her parents and deal with her step-brother.

She tapped while saying:

Even though I care for people and am able to help them through difficulties, I may consider having a little bit of fun for myself as well.

Even though I don't feel supported by anyone, and this is showing up as a pain in my back, I can accept and love all of me and deserve some pleasure in life.

Even though I feel as though I have to work all the time without enjoying any pleasures, I know it doesn't have to be like this, I can have my cake and eat it, too.

We decided to wind the session down at that point. After 60 minutes of tapping, Alison said that her feelings of rage had lessened a lot and that the pain in her back and shoulder had reduced. She also said that after all the money she had spent on alternative therapies over the past few years, she had never experienced as much relief as she had with EFT. Best of all, the EFT worked in a remarkably short space of time!

A few weeks later Alison reported that she was quite happy with the way the session had gone and that her back was much more comfortable. She added that she received a pleasant side effect of feeling calmer than she had ever felt in her life.

❊ ❊ ❊

As long as your subconscious mind has a reason for holding onto anger, it can be difficult if not impossible to dissolve. A leading reason for justifying anger and unforgiveness is the notion that if we forgive someone for something unforgivable, we're condoning what he or she did. Worse, we're encouraging that person to repeat the action or do something worse.

When It's Impossible to Forgive

by Cathleen Campbell

Often the concept of forgiveness is distasteful or seemingly impossible because it conveys a sense that what the offender did would be accepted or allowed without an apology, or that forgiveness would somehow signal to the offender that he or she could repeat the offense. We want the people who hurt us to acknowledge that pain, to convey their deep sorrow, and finally convince us that they will never again put us in such misery. Since our feelings are so strong, we believe we must be right and if we can't be right then not only must we be wrong but our pain would then be wrong, too. In such a state it's impossible to see that both parties could actually be right, or that perhaps there's some grey area in which no one is fully wrong. To comprehend and acknowledge all of this while in an acute state of pain is simply too much to bear.

But when we suspend judgment and simply tap for release, all sorts of new and interesting ideas begin to come to the surface. Since we are not asking ourselves to agree that something horribly wrong is now miraculously okay, our guard doesn't go up as firm and fast.

Shifting from the unproductive cycle of "they're wrong and I'm right" allows us to release our feelings of injustice. Sometimes the shifts can be so quick and dramatic that instead of maintaining the pain or grudge, a sense of understanding redefines the entire problem and we end up seeing the offender as the real victim!

Most often, though, asking our subconscious to help our conscious mind with understanding gives us new insights that allow us to slowly dissolve the pain. Even better, it helps us create new tactics with which to handle the situation. In situations that are ongoing, such as having to be around an offensive coworker or a family member, bringing new understanding into the equation gives us a new perspective from which to create the new reality we so dearly wish to live.

❊ ❊ ❊

Here's a report from EFT practitioner Stefan Gonick on this important issue.

Letting Go of Anger that Feels Necessary
by Stefan Gonick

I worked with three clients recently who had anger issues for which EFT tapping didn't initially help much at all. In each case, the person was angry about a serious offense that happened a very long time ago. There was nothing to be done or even said to the offending person, and in one case the offender had died. These clients were aware that the offenders from long ago were not being affected at all by their anger and that they were the only ones suffering. However, neither these realizations nor EFT relieved their anger.

When this happened with the first client, we were stuck for a while, but then I had a flash of intuition. I asked my client whether she felt that letting go of her anger would mean that the other person would somehow "get away with" what he did. A light bulb went on in her mind and she agreed.

She subconsciously felt that her anger was, in a cosmic justice sort of way, keeping the other person "accountable" for what he did. She was afraid that if she let go of her anger, it would mean that what he did to her "didn't matter" and he would "get away with it" without any consequences. The dilemma was that she herself was only person actually being affected by her anger, but it felt as though letting go of it would be to his benefit. So, we tapped on:

Even though he'll get away with what he did if I don't stay angry...

Even though he won't be accountable without my anger...

Even though my anger matters regarding what he did to me...

Later in the tapping we included affirming phrases like:

I release him to the Universe...

He is subject to his own karma...

I choose peace for myself...

After a several rounds of this nature, my client's anger disappeared and she felt great relief and peace around the issue.

After encountering this same situation with the next two clients in a row, I felt that this insight might be helpful to others, and it was. So, if you find yourself having a hard time relieving your anger through tapping, look deeper within to see if issues of "cosmic justice" are getting in your way.

❋ ❋ ❋

Australian EFT practitioner Angie Muccillo describes an EFT exercise that has widespread uses. The basic idea is to tap while you listen to your body in a unique way and let it tell you about the real issues underlying your pain. Along the way, you may discover metaphors that make core issues obvious or that help you understand just where your anger, discomfort, dissatisfaction, frustration, and pain are really coming from. If you haven't ever had a meaningful two-way conversation with your body, now's the time to begin.

What Your Aching Body Has to Say

by Angie Muccillo

You complain about your body—that damn shoulder, those bung knees, your sore back, that creaky neck—but how about giving your body a chance to complain about you? I wonder what it would have to say.

The purpose of this exercise is to give your painful body parts a chance to voice their point of view and express their pain and hurt while giving you a chance to really listen and take note. In this exercise, you will be paying attention to your aching, screaming body parts. This is an exercise in "in-tuition" or learning from within. It involves tuning in to your body and learning what it needs by listening to how it feels.

Communicating with your body in this way can re-establish or strengthen your connection to it. Sometimes we spend so much time complaining about our pain (either silently or aloud) that we forget to stop and listen for the message in the pain. Once we understand what our shoulder is angry about, for example, we can release it with EFT.

Let's see what a typical shoulder has to say. If you have a shoulder complaint of any sort, do your shoulder a favor and tap along. Simply tap the EFT points continuously as you read this script and borrow the benefits from this shoulder complaint. This is one uptight shoulder!

A Word From Your Shoulder Complaint

Hi, it's me, your shoulder. Yes, that's right. *remember me?* It's nice to be heard *finally!* Where do I begin? I've tried and tried to get your attention over and over again but you just won't listen to me. I have sent you repeated pain signals and messages but you ignore all my warnings and push on despite them. What's that all about? I don't understand why I have to get so red and angry to be heard. It's the only time you acknowledge me—and when you do, all I get is condemned. "That damn shoulder!" you cry. I feel like hunching over every time you hurl abuse at me. How do you think that makes me feel?

You complain about me. Well, you know what? I've got a few complaints of my own. I've been carrying your load and burdens all these years and what sort of appreciation do I get? *None!* To be honest, I am fed up and angry with you for treating me so badly. I've been supporting you all these years but I'm cracking and crumbling under the pressure. All I want is to know that I am doing a good job. Just the slightest acknowledgment would do. Some positive attention for a change would be greatly appreciated.

But you keep saying "yes" when you mean "no." I'm sick and tired of it. I wish you would follow your "no's" for a change. But because you don't follow your "no's," you always end up over-committing yourself and working too long and too hard and you don't even enjoy it most of the time. Then you take it all out on me and complain incessantly about how I bother you and what a pain I am and how I stop you from doing what you need to do. I just tighten up more and more every time I hear you say yes to something you don't want to do or be or have. I'm sick and tired of being tied up in knots all the time!

If you insist on carrying all those burdens and don't learn to say no when you mean no, then I'm going to have to say it for you by flaring up and firing a few more pain signals your way. I might even freeze right up so you can't move and then you'll be forced to stop what you are doing right there and then. I know that may seem a little harsh but that way you might get the message that I'm overworked and overtired and deserve a holiday!! Here's the deal. I'll rush you a load of those feel good chemicals you like so much, just as soon as you relax and give me a break! Deal?

Here are some step-by-step guidelines for writing your own script—How to "Take Note" of Your Complaints:

Step 1. Choose a physical complaint, and ask your complaint to state its own complaints.

Step 2. Invite your aching body part to speak up. Ask for the loudest complaint to come forward and deal with this one first.

Step 3. Focus on the area of your body you would like to heal—shoulder, neck, back, stomach—and ask it to tell you how it feels. Encourage your chosen body part to express any complaints and upsets openly and honestly and without holding back. Listen carefully and write down everything you are being told, take note of every complaint, every unheard request and every upset. You are at the service of your body here. Your job is simply to take note. Allow yourself to be creative in the process.

Step 4. Once you have finished your script, read it aloud and either tap continuously on the EFT points or rub the sore spot until you get to the end of the script and then use a Reminder Phrase at each point such as, "this (name of body part) complaint."

Step 5. Write a reply to your complaint in the form of a Self Care Plan. This is your chance to address your body's complaints. Write to your complaint or simply talk to it about your intentions to address its concerns. You may want to start by acknowledging its complaints and showing empathy for what it is experiencing. You can then explain what you plan to do (what action you will take) to address these complaints. For example, a Self Care Plan for the above shoulder complaint might sound something like the letter below. Again tap along to borrow the benefits.

Dear Shoulder — Yes, I hear you loud and clear now that I've stopped and taken time out of my busy schedule to take note of how you feel about all this. I know I've been a pain to live with lately, but things are going to change now. Even though in the past I was guilty of not listening to you, from now on I vow to tune in to how you are feeling and do what is necessary to take care of it. As soon as I start to receive a pain signal from you, I will promise to stop and look at what I'm doing that is overloading you. I vow to take care, respect, praise, and appreciate you for your hard work.

Yes, you have carried me all this time and now I take the time to show my appreciation. How's this—I will ensure that you get a massage at least once a fortnight, or weekly if your complaining gets too loud. I will take your advice and start saying no when I mean no. *Even though I've been guilty of saying "yes" when I mean "no," I choose to follow my "no's" from now on.* I will take a long hard look at what I take on and whether it is in my best interest. I put you first and focus on getting balance back into my life so that you don't have to work so hard. Hey and guess what! I just went to see the boss and I've put in for 6 weeks off. Now does that sound like a "Self Care Plan" or what?

If you have difficulty tuning into to your body and you can't 'hear' the messages, try these little EFT Tune Ups:

Even though I can't tune in to what my body is trying to tell me, I choose to listen for the message in the pain.

Even though I'm so out of touch with my body's needs, I choose to practice listening and taking note of what my body is trying to tell me.

Even though until now I have neglected and ignored the messages from my body, I choose to pay more attention from now on.

The more you take note of your body's complaints and tap on these complaints, the less likely it is that your body will complain at all. You can apply this process to all your physical complaints, starting with the loudest ones first.

Using this technique regularly may lead to pain reduction. It can also be used in a preventative manner by helping you stay in tune with your body and giving it what it needs for optimum health, whether it is better nutrition, more rest, more exercise, recovery time, letting go of certain obligations, cutting back work hours, increasing recreation time, increasing creative pursuits, or other factors that are there, in your body, waiting to be discovered.

❆ ❆ ❆

Here are some innovative approaches to chronic pain by Sangeeta Bhagwat from India. These same ideas can be useful for a wide variety of ailments. For those not familiar with paracetamol, which Sangeeta mentions in her report, it is the nonprescription painkiller known in the U.S. as acetaminophen (Tylenol).

EFT and Skillful Metaphors for Rheumatoid Arthritis Pain

by Sangeeta Bhagwat

I have been working with Mrs. J for her rheumatoid arthritis (RA) symptoms. RA pain is constant and terrible. As she had tried several allopathic (conventional) and Ayervedic (traditional Indian) medicines over the years, her homeopath asked her to avoid taking any medicines for about 15 to 20 days, to allow her body to detoxify. She continued her painkillers and a sleeping pill.

One day, her pain was highly unbearable, so she asked me to try EFT. She was complaining of severe pain in her shoulders. I first did one round using,

> *Even though I have this unbearable pain in my shoulders, I deeply and completely love, forgive and accept myself.*

She reported a reduction in her level of intensity from 8 to 7½ out of 10. I then asked her to describe the pain, asking her whether it had a color or texture. She replied that it was dark grey and like a sticky liquid.

So I started tapping on her with the following setup:

> *Even though I have this dark grey, sticky pain weighing down my shoulders, I choose to drain it away.*

While I was tapping, I told her to imagine a tube draining away this pain, while she repeated *"drain away"* at each point. Two rounds reduced her level of intensity to 2 out of 10.

I asked her to describe the pain again. She said it was now dark and thick. So while tapping at the Karate Chop point, we used:

> *Even though I have this stubborn, dark and sticky pain in my shoulders, I apply heat to it so that it*

becomes thinner and can drain away easily. I drain away this remaining pain.

The pain subsided. I worked on some more underlying emotional issues and gave her homework rounds to do.

After a few days, she again called with severe shoulder pain. When asked to describe it, she called the pain "four huge boulders." So I used:

Even though these four heavy boulders are weighing me down, I choose to break them with a laser gun.

That did not work, so I changed it to:

Even though these four boulders are weighing me down, I choose to hammer them to pieces,

with "hammer" as the Reminder Phrase. Immediately, she felt that the boulders had shattered to pieces and the pain had "rolled away."

She then stood up with some difficulty and said that the pain had dropped to around her hips. When asked to describe it, she said it was like a string of heavy rocks around her hip. So I used:

Even though I have this money belt of painful rocks around my hip, I deeply and completely love, forgive and accept myself.

There was only a marginal movement in her level of intensity.

I felt that she was reluctant to let go of the pain, so I changed the setup to

Even though this pain is terrible, I don't want to change. I am used to it and don't want to let go.

After tapping one shortcut round of this, I changed the setup to:

Even though I don't want to let go of these ten rocks I have around my hip, perhaps I could let go of just one.

After this round, she said three rocks had fallen off. So I repeated the setup with seven *remaining rocks.* Shortly there was only one left. So I made the setup:

I can keep this one rock, as I am so used to it.

However, on completing the round, there were no "rocks" left!

With regular tapping, Mrs. J. was gradually able to reduce pain and swelling. She reduced her medication to one painkiller a day and no sleeping pills. Her homeopath also started treatment. After about two weeks, he told her to consider dropping her painkiller and if necessary, using a paracetamol instead.

She was highly troubled by this as she felt that she was dependent on the painkiller and without it, the pain would be unbearable. We discussed the possible side effects of painkillers and I suggested we try tapping in the paracetamol as a substitute. She agreed.

So we did one round using:

Even though I think that only the prescription painkiller can provide relief from terrible pain, taking the paracetamol will prove to be equally effective for me.

Happily, she made the transition very smoothly and says that the paracetamol worked as effectively as the strong painkiller she had been using. We plan to tap away her dependence on this pill after a couple of days. I think this may be a useful way to taper people off addictive and strong medications.

In our last session, after some discussion, she felt that she was facing an internal battle, where there was a part of her that wanted to return to complete health and another that felt attached to the disease as it had served in getting her attention from others and kept family tied to her. (Fear of rejection is one of her major underlying emotional issues).

I asked her to give this defiant part of herself a name and appearance. She called it "Inflexibility" and said it looked like a shadowy image of herself. We tapped for:

Even though Inflexibility does not want me to change and be well, I deeply and completely love, forgive, and accept myself.

She felt that the image was shrinking in size, until it looked like a small girl with two plaits, wearing a sari. Unsurprisingly, it reminded her of herself as a child. We next tapped on:

Even though Inflexibility has been staging this scary drama where I suffer a great deal of pain and I allowed myself to be conned by this play, I deeply and completely love, forgive and accept myself,

This was followed by:

There is nothing to fear, I am safe and well.

In her mind, the little girl burst into tears, so I told her to hug her and tapped:

Even though she scared me, she meant no harm. She was doing the best she knew. I deeply and completely love, forgive and accept her.

At the end of this session, Mrs. J. was feeling substantially lighter, happier and stronger. She felt optimistic about improvement and is now more motivated to fight her symptoms. Clearly, there is more work required, but there has certainly been noticeable improvement in her. I think the combination of EFT and homeopathy is proving to be highly effective for reducing her symptoms, in a relatively short time.

Update: I have been in regular touch with Mrs. J. over the past months. She is one of the most consistent and persistent tappers that I know. When I wrote the above report nine months ago, her Rheumatoid Factor was 72. She has been taking homeopathic treatment and continues with extensive tapping. In December 2007, seven months after she started tapping, her Rheumatoid Factor was down to 4. Her homeopathic doctor believes that she no longer has RA and her present symptoms are likely caused by cold weather and unresolved emotional issues.

Mrs. J. has unearthed many such emotional issues and has been working on various incidents and issues in her life. With the help of a pendulum and substance sensitivity charts, we found her to be sensitive to calcium and iron. After tapping for the same, she feels that her supplements are finally beginning to show a positive impact on her strength and energy. She has often noticed pain relief while tapping for issues related to forgiveness, rigidity and resistance to change. On many occasions, Mrs. J. requires the Collarbone Breathing Technique for Psychological Reversal.

Mrs. J. continues to have frequent episodes of stubborn pain and skin problems. While there are many emotional and physical problems yet to be healed, she has already made incredible progress, and her commitment and faith in EFT is unshaken.

※ ※ ※

12

Freedom from Pain
through Forgiveness

We may intellectually understand that forgiveness is a good thing, but realizing that same fact emotionally can be a challenge. This is true even after we give ourselves vivid demonstrations of how closely our pain is tied to anger, the way Caroline, the school bus driver, did. We may even practice a religion that emphasizes forgiveness. Yet some of us would rather keep the pain forever than let go of the anger.

If this is your situation, you'll find it difficult if not impossible to tap through a Setup Phrase that forgives the cause of your pain, such as:

Even though this pain gets worse when I think about my boss and how he treated me, I forgive him now.

Even though this pain gets worse whenever I think of how my sister betrayed me, I choose to forgive her and get on with my life.

Even though it's hard to forgive him for what he did, I know that holding on to my anger only makes the pain worse, so I choose to forgive him now and let the pain go.

Even though I blame myself for this pain, I love and forgive myself anyway.

Forgiveness comes in many shades and, for some, forgiveness is truly impossible—at least for the time being. Some clients dig in their heels at the mere mention of "forgiving that bastard" and will go no further if forgiveness is the goal.

Add "Understanding"

Fortunately, the word "understand" carries less emotional baggage than the word "forgive," so adding it to the Setup Phrase can help ease the transition from guilt or blame toward forgiveness and release.

Even though this pain gets worse when I think about my boss and how he treated me, I understand how this all happened.

Even though this pain gets worse whenever I think of how my sister betrayed me, I understand why she did what she did.

Even though it's hard to forgive him for what he did, I know that holding on to my anger only makes the pain worse, so I choose to understand his situation now and let the pain go.

Even though I blame myself for this pain, I understand why I did what I did, which was the best I could do at the time.

This substitution can help you switch mental gears and look at any situation differently. Whenever this happens while you're telling an old, familiar story, it's a clear indication that your energy blocks are clearing. Any "cognitive shift," as psychologists call it, is a sign that EFT is working.

Release "a Little" Anger

Total forgiveness can seem like an impossible homework assignment. Fortunately, the simple strategy of giving up a little anger can go a long way toward releasing the rest. Some ways to do this are to project your release of anger far into the future or to make the whole project indefinite.

…I choose to know that I can some day release this anger…

…I might someday, perhaps, forgive him a little…

This all sounds very vague, but it replaces a flat "it's never going to happen" with the possibility of a future transformation.

Here is an important report from Dr. Patricia Carrington, who calls her elegant application of incremental EFT the "one-percent solution." That's a great name for a highly effective technique.

Using EFT for Forgiveness: the One-percent Solution

by Dr. Patricia Carrington

I can't tell you how often people have told me that they simply cannot conceive of forgiving some other person for destructive acts that person has done—even if they use EFT for this problem. They feel that to do this would be paying mere lip service to the concept of "forgiveness." It would not come from their heart.

I agree that the act of "forgiveness" is all too often a pretense entered into by a person who feels obliged to "forgive" someone (or fate), perhaps for religious or ethical reasons. To truly forgive, especially when one feels resentment, fear, or anger about a "wrong" that has been done to self or others, is one of the most difficult and "unintuitive" things that we can do.

The reason for this may be the fact that the act of forgiving is not an act at all in any real sense. When it happens it does so by default, as we let go of resentment against the other party along with the desire to punish.

Webster's New International Dictionary and the *Oxford Dictionary of the English Language* both define the verb *to forgive* as "to give up resentment against or the desire to punish; to stop being angry with; to pardon." It is quite clear that their definitions of forgiveness refer to the result of *letting go* of anger or resentment or desire for revenge. Forgiveness, then, is basically an *absence* of these negative emotions.

This makes for difficulty, however, when we attempt to use EFT to create forgiveness because it is much more difficult for people or animals to let go of something than it is for them to hold on to it. Ask someone, for example, to place a book on a table, and more than likely (if they have no particular reason for not doing so) they will find it easy to comply with your request for they are being asked to do a direct and simple act.

However, ask that same person to "let go" of a book they might already be holding and they may well resist that request, or at least hesitate to carry it out until they give considerable thought to the consequences. They will probably consider possible outcomes that come to their mind and will try to decide whether it is safe and advantageous for them to let go of the book. Perhaps it will fall upon the floor and get damaged. Maybe the person will be "pushed around" or otherwise manipulated by you if he or she complies with this request. The result is that this person may be reluctant to let go of the book.

I am reminded of the way newborn infants show such a powerful grasp reflex. They can hold on with enormous strength to a finger or object within reach and not let go of it for a long time—sometimes their fingers have to be pried loose from the object. This grasp reflex may well be due to some inherited instinct that helped newborn humans to survive when we were tree-dwelling primates. It is likely that newborns had to be able to grasp onto their mothers or onto a tree branch to protect against a disastrous fall.

Whatever the reason, the fact is that it is usually easier for us to hold on to something that it is to let go of that same thing, and because of our use of language, we have a strong tendency to hold on to remembered wrongs and seemingly cannot pry ourselves loose from thoughts about "justice" and "punishment" for such wrongs. We cling to such thoughts tenaciously for long periods of time, sometimes for a lifetime, and it is not surprising that we hear stories of vendettas that carry on from generation to generation in certain cultures, where a revenge motive actually controls the lives of the people caught in it.

How then can we bring about "forgiveness," which basically involves a *letting go* of resentment and giving up of the wish for revenge, even with the use of EFT?

Because forgiveness is actually something that happens automatically when resentment, anger, revenge and a desire to punish have been relinquished, I am going to suggest a way in which EFT can be used to lessen or eliminate resentment and the punishment motive, thereby creating the natural state of forgiveness which is, in fact, an absence of the need for revenge.

Since there is much reluctance in people to let go of resentment and the need for retribution, I have found it is far more productive to approach this matter in an indirect manner, little by little. One way I have found extremely effective is to break up the revenge motive into tiny manageable pieces. I call this the "Divide and Conquer" tactic. Here's how it works.

Suppose that one person has been deeply hurt another person in the past. If you ask Person A to "forgive" Person B, it seems impossible at first. Even if you ask her or him to "let go" of any resentment they have toward the other person, it still tends to feel impossible. How, they reason, can someone just let go of resentment if they've been deeply hurt?

A way to get around this trap, one which I find to be extraordinarily effective, is to **break up** the "letting go" process into tiny chunks, so that you *prove* to yourself that your conviction that it's impossible to let go of your resentment isn't true, that resentment *can* be let go of in little pieces—which of course paves the way for a much greater letting go to come.

When you formulate your EFT statement, end the statement by a Choice to "let go of only one percent" of your resentment. You can even add the phrase "and keep all the rest of it" if you wish. Here is how this statement might look in practice.

Even though I'm outraged at what he did, I choose to let go of one percent of my anger against him.

Even though I'm furious about what she did, I choose to release one percent of the rage I feel toward her.

If you use this "one-percent" solution, you will probably have no trouble letting go of such a ridiculously small portion of your resentment. After all, it is not much to ask of yourself to give up one percent of it, and you are still allowed to retain most of your righteous anger!

However—and here is the secret in this approach —if you are able truly to let go of one percent of your resentment, anger, or desire to punish, then you will be in a very different state of mind than you were before. Something that seemed impossible will suddenly become possible, even if on a very small scale, and by letting it happen at all, you have actually opened a door to letting go of your resentments totally. A little release is always a big release. You will now have abandoned a deeply entrenched belief, a certainty that you *cannot* under any circumstances let go of your resentment!

I have many times seen this simple strategy result in a person's ability to entertain the *possibility* of letting go of *all* of their resentment. Once relinquishing a desire for revenge is seen as possible, the road has been cleared for you to release your entire resentment/punishment motive. When you let go of your tenacious hold on the conviction that "justice must be done at any cost," and punishment must be meted out for you to be at rest, you finally will be at rest. You will have lifted a tremendous emotional burden from yourself, and you'll be able to move ahead constructively with your life.

You may decide that you don't want to see that person again or put yourself in that kind of situation again, or you may decide to do so, according to rational decision. Either way, you are now free to choose what is really best for you. This is because the emotional charge has been removed from the situation. Now you will have "forgiven" that person in the true sense of that word. The revenge motive will have evaporated, and because unforgiveness depends on that motive, it too will have melted away. You will have forgiven this person or circumstance or fate in the true sense of the word, and can go on from there to build a new relationship or other better relationships or whatever you desire.

I strongly recommend the "one-percent solution" when the need to forgive is resistant to any other approach.

※ ※ ※

EFT Gratitude Protocol

I'm big on gratitude. There is much to be grateful for and when we adopt that state many interesting doors open. For example, filling the mind with gratitude leaves little room for unforgiveness, so if you're having trouble letting go of anger, blame, frustration, and other unforgiving emotions, try this approach. It's both easy and comfortable, and it can ease the transition toward complete forgiveness.

Angie Muccillo gives us some specific ways to apply gratitude to EFT, but her idea can be applied to anything.

Tapping on Gratitude with EFT

by Angie Muccillo

Here's a simple little EFT protocol with the potential to increase EFT's effectiveness.

Are you grateful to EFT? I definitely am. I am grateful for not only the many positive effects it has had on my life personally, but also the many wondrous changes and healing I see in others as a result of using EFT. I think most people who have used EFT and achieved some degree of success with their personal and emotional issues have felt and expressed gratitude for what EFT has done for them. We have many documented accounts of these on the EFT website and in our clinics and offices worldwide.

EFT instructor Carol Tuttle recommends we tap on everything we are grateful for in our lives, as a way of focusing on what we have or want to attract more of. So I thought why not add EFT to that list? In essence, if we want to attract more success with our use of EFT, let's express our gratitude for it, like anything else. Carol also states, "Gratitude is one of the highest states of emotion we can experience." If we tap on our gratitude for EFT, we are focusing on our highest thoughts of EFT and placing our attention and thoughts on what we are grateful that EFT is doing for us. In other words we use the EFT affirmation to affirm EFT!

Tap on Gratitude for EFT

The idea is simply to use the EFT Gratitude Protocol at the end (or beginning) of a tapping session with a round or two of statements focused on our gratitude towards EFT. I think giving thanks to EFT is a kind of pleasant and harmonious way to open or close a tapping session whether it is with a practitioner or on your own.

Whether the session has completely resolved your issues or not, inserting the Gratitude Protocol at the end, may set a positive scene for future tapping and perhaps help build a bridge to the next session. I would also recommend using the Gratitude Protocol routinely as a daily or homework exercise or when you feel "stuck."

EFT Gratitude Statements:

Tap the EFT points while repeating each statement:

I am deeply and completely grateful for EFT.

I am deeply and completely grateful for releasing these emotions with EFT.

I am deeply and completely grateful for the ease with which EFT is helping me to release my fears, phobias, and traumatic memories.

I am deeply and completely grateful to EFT for relieving my back/shoulder pain.

I am deeply and completely grateful for the ease with which EFT is helping me to release my addictions.

I am deeply and completely grateful that I have EFT to help me release my pain and suffering.

I am deeply and completely grateful for the ease with which EFT works for me each and every time.

I am deeply and completely grateful that I have a tool to help me calm down whenever I need it.

I am deeply and completely grateful for the positive changes EFT has helped me make in my life.

I am deeply and completely grateful for the many benefits I am receiving from using EFT daily.

I am deeply and completely grateful for the positive impact EFT is having on my life and those around me.

I am deeply and completely grateful for the peace and calm EFT has brought into my life.

I am deeply and completely grateful to EFT for improving the quality of my life.

I am deeply and completely grateful I have discovered this wonderful tool!

These are just a few suggestions. I am sure there's a lot of gratitude out there for EFT! Let's hear it and share it. As a general rule write your statements as though your EFT goals have already been achieved.

This protocol may also be useful when EFT "doesn't appear to be working" or you feel "stuck" or frustrated. While there are many one-minute wonders in EFT, as we know, some issues do take time to break down and in the process we may find ourselves getting frustrated, overwhelmed even unappreciative and forgetful of the progress we have actually made. We can use this protocol to help break free from some of these barriers by switching our thinking to what we are grateful for instead.

We can use the Choices method to install gratitude.

Example Set Ups:

Even though EFT isn't working for my back pain yet, I choose to be grateful to EFT for helping me release these emotions and for all the healing I have achieved so far.

Even though I don't get the same results as Mary did, I choose to be grateful I have a tool to help me calm down whenever I need it.

Even though I'm sick of tapping and don't seem to be getting anywhere, I am grateful for the positive changes EFT has helped me make in my life.

What are you grateful for when it comes to EFT? Write your list of gratitude statements and tap on them regularly.

✿ ✿ ✿

In Conclusion...

Whether you're working with yourself, your spouse or partner, your children, a friend or relative, a client, a patient, or a favorite pet, EFT is a powerful tool for the relief of all types of pain and discomfort. I hope you will join me in exploring its powerful benefits. Master what's in these pages and you will never view healing the same way again. Together we will build within you a bridge to the land of personal peace. Once built, this bridge will become a lifetime skill that you can use to spread emotional freedom and joy from yourself to others. And it's permanent. Like gold, it doesn't rust or tarnish or become obsolete. It will always be there for you.

The End

EFT Glossary

The following terms have specific meanings in EFT. They are referred to in some of the reports included here and are often mentioned in EFT reports.

Acupoints. Acupuncture points which are sensitive points along the body's meridians. Acupoints can be stimulated by acupuncture needles or, in acupressure, by massage or tapping. EFT is an acupressure tapping technique.

Art of Delivery. The sophisticated presentation of EFT that uses imagination, intuition, and humor to quickly discover and treat the underlying causes of pain and other problems. The art of delivery goes far beyond Mechanical EFT.

Aspects are "issues within issues," different facets or pieces of a problem that are related but separate. When new aspects appear, EFT can seem to stop working. In truth, the original EFT treatment continues to work while the new aspect triggers a new set of symptoms. In some cases,

278 EFT for Back Pain

many aspects of a situation or problem each require their own EFT treatment. In others, only a few do.

Basic Formula. See Mechanical EFT.

Basic Recipe. A four-step treatment consisting of Setup phrase, Sequence (tapping on acupoints in order), 9-Gamut Treatment, and Sequence. This was the original EFT protocol.

Borrowing Benefits. When you tap with or on behalf of another person, your own situation improves, even though you aren't tapping for your own situation. This happens in one-on-one sessions, in groups, and when you perform surrogate or proxy tapping. The more you tap for others, the more your own life improves.

Chasing the Pain. After applying EFT, physical discomforts can move to other locations and/or change in intensity or quality. A headache described as a sharp pain behind the eyes at an intensity of 8 might shift to dull throb in back of the head at an intensity of 7 (or 9, or 3 or any other intensity level). Moving pain is an indication that EFT is working. Keep "chasing the pain" with EFT and it will usually go to zero or some low number. In the process, emotional issues behind the discomforts are often successfully treated.

Chi. *Chi,* or energy, flows through and around every living being. It is said to regulate spiritual, emotional, mental, and physical balance and to be influenced by *yin* (the receptive, feminine force) and *yang* (the active masculine force). These forces, which are complementary opposites, are in constant motion. When *yin* and *yang* are balanced, they work together with the natural flow of *chi* to help the body achieve and maintain health. *Chi* moves through the body along invisible pathways, or channels, called meridians Traditional Chinese Medicine identifies 20 meridians along which chi or vital energy flows or circulate through to all parts of the body. Acupoints along the meridians can be stimulated to improve the flow of *Chi* and, in EFT, to resolve emotional issues.

Choices Method. Dr. Patricia Carrington's method for inserting positive statements and solutions into Setup and Reminder Phrases.

Core Issues. Core issues are deep, important underlying emotional imbalances, usually created in response to traumatic events. A core issue is truly the crux of the problem, its root or heart. Core issues are not always obvious but careful detective work can often uncover them, and once discovered, they can be broken down into specific events and handled routinely with EFT.

Generalization Effect. When related issues are neutralized with EFT, they often take with them issues that are related in the person's mind. In this way, several issues can be resolved even though only one is directly treated.

Global. While the term "global" usually refers to something that is universal or experienced worldwide, In EFT it refers to problems, especially in Setup phrases, that are vague and not specific.

Intensity Meter. The 0-to-10 scale that measures pain, discomfort, anger, frustration, and every other physical or emotional symptom. Intensity can also be indicated with gestures, such as hands held close together (small discomfort) or wide apart (large discomfort).

Mechanical EFT. EFT's Basic Formula consists of tapping on the Karate Chop point or Sore Spot while saying three times, "Even though I have this ___[problem]___, I fully and complete accept myself" (Setup phrase), followed by three rounds of tapping the Sequence of EFT acupoints in order, with an appropriate Reminder Phrase.

Meridians. Invisible channels or pathways through which energy or *Chi* flows in the body. The eight primary meridians pass through five pairs of vital organs, and twelve secondary meridians network to the extremities. The basic premise of EFT is that the cause of every negative emotion and most physical symptoms is a block or disruption in the flow of *Chi,* or energy, along one or more of the meridians.

Movie Technique, or Watch a Movie Technique. In this process you review in your mind, as though it were a movie, a bothersome specific event. When intensity comes up, stop and tap on that intensity. When the intensity subsides, continue in your mind with the story. This method has been a mainstay in the tool box of many EFT practitioners. It may be the most-often used EFT technique of all. For a full description, see www.emofree.com/tutorial/tutorcthree.htm

Personal Peace Procedure. An exercise in which you clear problems and release core issues by writing down, as quickly as possible, as many bothersome events from your life that you can remember. Try for at least 50 or 100. Give each event a title, as though it is a book or movie. When the list is complete, begin tapping on the largest issues. Eliminating at least one uncomfortable memory per day (a very conservative schedule) removes at least 90 unhappy events in three months. If you work through two or three per day, it's 180 or 270. For details, see www.emofree.com/tutorial/tutormthirteen.htm.

Reminder Phrase. A word, phrase, or sentence that helps the mind focus on the problem being treated. It is used in combination with acupoint tapping.

Setup phrase, or Setup. An opening statement said at the beginning of each EFT treatment which defines and helps neutralize the problem. In EFT, the standard Setup phrase is, "Even though I have this _____, I fully and completely accept myself."

Story Technique, or Tell a Story Technique. Narrate or tell the story out loud of a specific event dealing with trauma, grief, anger, etc., and stop to tap whenever the story becomes emotionally intense. Each of the stopping points represents another aspect of the issue that, on occasion, will take you to even deeper issues. This technique is identical to the Movie Technique except that in the Movie Technique, you simply watch past events unfold in your mind. In the Tell a Story Technique, you describe them out loud.

Surrogate or Proxy Tapping involves tapping on yourself on behalf of another person. The person can be present or not. Another way to perform surrogate or proxy tapping is to substitute a photograph, picture, or line drawing for the person and tap on that.

Tail-enders. The "yes, but" statements that create negative self-talk. When you state a goal or affirmation, tail-enders point the way to core issues.

Tearless Trauma Technique. This is another way of approaching an emotional problem in a gentle way. It involves having the client guess as to the emotional intensity of a past event rather than painfully re-live it mentally.

Writings on Your Walls. Limiting beliefs and attitudes that result from cultural conditioning or family attitudes, these are often illogical and harmful yet very strong subconscious influences.

Yin and Yang. See *Chi,* above.

EFT Resources

For details about EFT, including our free download-able manual in 19 languages, information about ordering our DVDs, referrals to EFT practitioners, online tutorials, books and e-books, hundreds of reports describing EFT in action, and other helpful information, visit www.emofree.com.

Index

A world of wellness at your fingertips!

To see more books in this series of authorized EFT guides, including....

The EFT Manual
EFT for Weight Loss
EFT for Fibromyalgia and Chronic Fatigue
EFT for the Highly Sensitive Temperament
EFT for Golf
EFT for Love Relationships
EFT for Abundance
EFT for Post Traumatic Stress Syndrome
EFT for Procrastination
EFT for Back Pain

Go to www.EFTBookShelf.com